Medical Radiology

Radiation Oncology

Series editors
Luther W. Brady
Stephanie E. Combs
Jiade J. Lu

Honorary Editors
Hans-Peter Heilmann
Michael Molls

For further volumes:
http://www.springer.com/series/4353

Jonathan Strauss · William Small
Gayle E. Woloschak

Editors

Breast Cancer Biology for the Radiation Oncologist

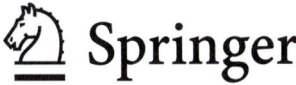

Editors

Jonathan Strauss
Department of Radiation Oncology
Northwestern University
Chicago, IL
USA

William Small
Department of Radiation Oncology,
   Stritch School of Medicine, Cardinal Bernardin
   Cancer Center
Loyola University Chicago
Maywood, IL
USA

Gayle E. Woloschak
Department of Radiology
Northwestern University Feinberg
   School of Medicine
Chicago, IL
USA

ISSN 0942-5373   ISSN 2197-4187   (electronic)
Medical Radiology
ISBN 978-3-662-52074-1   ISBN 978-3-642-31220-5   (eBook)
DOI 10.1007/978-3-642-31220-5

Springer Heidelberg New York Dordrecht London
© Springer-Verlag Berlin Heidelberg 2015
Softcover reprint of the hardcover 1st edition 2015

Printed on acid-free paper

Springer-Verlag GmbH Berlin Heidelberg is part of Springer Science+Business Media (www.springer.com)

Contents

Contributors

Mashrafi Ahmed Saint Joseph Hospital, Chicago, USA

Sara E. Barnato Northwestern University, Chicago, IL, USA

William J. Gradishar Northwestern University, Chicago, IL, USA

Camille Green Department of Radiation Oncology, UMDNJ-RWJMS, Cancer Institute of New Jersey, New Brunswick, NJ, USA

Bruce G. Haffty Department of Radiation Oncology, UMDNJ-RWJMS, Cancer Institute of New Jersey, New Brunswick, NJ, USA

Sanaz A. Jansen Frederick National Laboratory for Cancer Research, Mouse Cancer Genetics Program, National Cancer Institute, Frederick, MD, USA

Atif J. Khan Department of Radiation Oncology, UMDNJ-RWJMS, Cancer Institute of New Jersey, New Brunswick, NJ, USA

William T. Leslie Rush University Medical Center, Chicago, USA

Jian Jian Li Department of Radiation Oncology, University of California Davis, Sacramento, CA, USA

Dhara MacDermed St. Charles Cancer Treatment Center, Bend, OR, USA

Clodia Osipo Molecular Biology Program, Loyola University Chicago, Maywood, IL, USA; Department of Pathology/Oncology Institute, Loyola University Chicago, Maywood, IL, USA; Department of Microbiology and Immunology, Loyola University Chicago, Maywood, IL, USA

Kinnari Pandya Molecular Biology Program, Loyola University Chicago, Maywood, IL, USA

Bryan M. Rabatic Department of Radiation Oncology, Georgia Regents University, Augusta, USA

Ruta Rao Rush University Medical Center, Chicago, USA

Biological Subtypes of Breast Cancer

Sara E. Barnato and William J. Gradishar

Contents

Abstract

Breast cancer is no longer thought of as a single disease, but rather as collection of subtypes characterized by molecular signatures. The use of gene array analysis has provided insights into the dominant driver pathways that effect individual tumors and translate into clinical manifestations of the disease, response to treatment and overall clinical outcome.

Breast cancer represents a heterogeneous group of diseases with various clinical presentations, responses to treatment, and outcomes. Several clinical factors affect prognosis, such as tumor size, nodal involvement, nuclear grade, histologic type, molecular markers, and surgical margins. Even taking these factors into account, there remains great variation in the behavior of breast cancer. The limitations of the prognostic value of these variables have underscored the rational for developing gene expression profiling of tumor tissue to try to further classify individual tumors to provide more reliable information regarding response to prognosis and treatment. Perou et al. (2000) proposed that the phenotypical diversity of breast tumors could also be associated with diverse gene expression patterns. To evaluate this, Perou et al. used cDNA microarrays to analyze genetic profiles and grouped genes based on their similar patterns of expression. Subsequently, Sorlie et al. (2001, 2003) demonstrated breast tumors can be divided into four distinct molecular subtypes: (i) luminal A, (ii) luminal B, (iii) HER2-type, and (iv) basal-like. Investigations of these subtypes in women with breast cancer have given insight into the heterogeneous biology and outcomes in patients with early-stage and locally advanced disease. These subtypes have subsequently been found to correlate with prognosis, response to systemic therapy, and locoregional recurrence.

S.E. Barnato · W.J. Gradishar (✉)
Northwestern University, 676 N. St. Clair,
Suite 850, Chicago, IL 60611, USA
e-mail: w-gradishar@northwestern.edu

J. Strauss et al. (eds.), *Breast Cancer Biology for the Radiation Oncologist*, Medical Radiology. Radiation Oncology,
DOI: 10.1007/174_2014_1043, © Springer-Verlag Berlin Heidelberg 2015
Published Online: 11 February 2015

1   Molecular Subtypes of Breast Cancer

The four distinct molecular subtypes are as follows: (i) luminal A, (ii) luminal B, (iii) HER2-type, and (iv) basal-like. The two luminal subtypes (luminal A and B) comprise most ER-positive breast cancers and are characterized by a high expression of hormone receptor (HR)-related genes. The HER2-enriched subtype is characterized by high expression of HER2-related and proliferation genes and low expression of HR-related genes (Sorlie et al. 2001, 2003; Sotiriou et al. 2003). The basal-like subtype is characterized by the absence of expression of hormonal and HER2 receptors and has a high expression of proliferation genes.

Until recently, strict tissue requirements, costs, complexity, and technical challenges have limited the application of gene expression profiling to clinical practice. Now, however, commercially available assays such as Oncotype DX® and MammaPrint® have become more widely used. Immunohistochemistry (IHC), using various biomarkers, has been used as a surrogate to the molecular subtypes. IHC is inexpensive, readily available, reliable, reproducible, and technically simple. Antibodies for estrogen receptor (ER), progesterone receptor (PR), HER2, cytokeratin 5/6 (CK 5/6), epidermal growth factor (EGFR), and Ki67 have been used to classify subtypes of breast cancer. Whether IHC analysis of tumor markers categorizes tumors identically to molecular subtyping is debatable.

Luminal A breast cancer is the most common subtype, accounting for 50–60 % of breast cancers. As previously mentioned, it is characterized by the expression of genes activated by the ER transcription factor that are typically expressed in the luminal epithelium lining the mammary ducts. It is also associated with a low expression of genes related to cell proliferation. The luminal A IHC profile is characterized by ER +/− PR expression, an absence of HER2 expression, a low rate of proliferation measured by Ki67 (suggested to be <14 %), and a low histological grade. While women with luminal A, early-stage breast cancer have the best prognosis and relatively low rates of local and regional relapses (Voduc et al. 2010), they frequently have bone as the first site of metastatic disease (Sihto et al. 2011).

Luminal B tumors make up between 10 and 20 % of all breast cancers. Compared to luminal A, they have a more aggressive phenotype, higher histological grade and proliferative index, and a worse prognosis. The pattern of distant relapse also differs, and although bone remains the most common site of recurrence (30 %), this subtype has a high recurrence rate in visceral sites such as the liver (13.8 %). Additionally, the survival from time of relapse is lower (1.6 years) compared to luminal A (2.2 years) (Kennecke et al. 2010). The main biological difference between the luminal A and B subtypes is an increase expression of proliferation genes. From the IHC standpoint, there have been attempts to differentiate between luminal A and luminal B using the protein expression of Ki67 as a possible marker (Cheang et al. 2009). The luminal A subtype has been defined as ER-positive/HER2-negative and low Ki67, while the luminal B subtype has tumors with ER-positive/HER2-negative and high Ki67 or ER-positive/HER2-positive. There are also approximately 6 % of luminal B subtype tumors that are ER-negative and HER2-negative. It is also important to note that the cutoff point for Ki67 has not been standardized. Since the prognosis of luminal B tumors is different compared with luminal A, an effort to identify biomarkers that distinguish between these two subgroups has been made.

HER2-positive breast cancers are characterized by the overexpression of the HER2 gene and genes related to cellular proliferation. These tumors are highly proliferative with approximately 75 % having a high histological grade and more than 40 % having p53 mutations. HER2-enriched tumors have a high rate of local recurrence (21 % vs. 8 % for luminal A); however, it is important to note that these data were obtained before the routine use of adjuvant trastuzumab so it is reasonable to assume the risk of local recurrence would be reduced with its use. Patients with HER2-overexpressing breast cancer have a higher frequency of developing brain metastases compared to other subtypes of breast cancer brain (Gabos et al. 2006), in addition to a higher rate of metastases to the liver and lung (Kennecke et al. 2010).

The basal-like subtype typically expresses genes present in normal breast myoepithelial cells, including cytokeratins CK5 and CK17, P-cadherin, CD44, and EGFR. Clinically, basal-like tumors are characterized by young age at diagnosis, greater frequency in African–American women, larger tumor size at diagnosis, high histological grade, and a high frequency of lymph node involvement. Basal-like tumors tend to have a high mitotic index and are associated with tumor necrosis. They behave in a clinically aggressive manner with a predominance of involvement in visceral organs, mainly lungs, central nervous system, and lymph nodes. Basal-like tumors typically, but not uniformly, lack expression of the three key receptors in breast cancers: ER, PR, and HER2 receptor overexpression. In clinical practice, the terms basal-like and triple negative are often interchanged; however, they are not synonymous. The majority of basal-like breast cancers have a triple-negative phenotype, and the vast majority of triple-negative cancers display a basal-like phenotype.

Park et al. (2012) evaluated characteristics and outcomes of patients according to molecular subtypes of breast cancer as classified by a panel of four biomarkers using IHC. They used ER, PR, HER2, and Ki-67 expression to categorize 1,066 breast cancer patients into the four subgroups. Demographics, recurrence patterns, and survival were retrospectively analyzed. In their study, luminal A, luminal B,

HER2-enriched, and basal-like tumors accounted for 53.1, 21.7, 9.0, and 16.2 % of cases, respectively. Luminal A tumors were well differentiated and had a higher expression of HR than luminal B. HER2-enriched tumors were associated with larger tumor size and higher frequency of nodal metastasis. Basal-like tumors were associated with younger age at diagnosis, larger primary tumor size, higher proliferation index (i.e., Ki67), poor differentiation, and frequent visceral metastases. In addition, by using IHC, they found similar recurrence patterns and survival outcomes consistent with subtyping by cDNA microarray. Molecular subtyping based on IHC remains a standard first step for informing treatment and surveillance strategies in breast cancer patients.

2   How Subtypes May Affect Response to Therapy?

The molecular subtypes of early-stage breast cancer have quite variable disease outcomes such that some patients are cured of their disease with standard therapy, while others develop rapid disease progression despite standard multimodal treatment. The molecular subtypes provide insight into the variable clinical outcomes in patients and may serve as prognostic tools and predictors of response to systemic adjuvant therapy.

A number of studies have explored the effect of the molecular subtype on both response to preoperative chemotherapy and survival (Bertucci et al. 2005; Rouzier et al. 2005; Rody et al. 2007; Carey et al. 2007; Goldstein et al. 2007; Guarneri et al. 2006; Fernandez-Morales et al. 2007; Sanchez-Munoz et al. 2008; Colleoni et al. 2008). These investigations have shown that the rate of pathologic complete response (pCR) in both breast tissue and axillary lymph nodes differs considerably among the molecular subtypes. The luminal A subtype had a very low rate of pCR (on average less than 10 %, 0–27 %) in patients treated with a variety of preoperative chemotherapy regimens. There was a high rate of pCR seen with the basal-like (on average 40 %, 10–80 %) and HER2-enriched subtypes (on average 40 %, 20–62 %). The luminal B subtype was associated with an intermediate rate of response (on average less than 20 %, 15–33 %).

The high rate of pCR observed with basal-like, and HER2-enriched tumors seem to contrast with the inferior survival of these patients. However, patients who have a pCR have superior survival regardless of their subtype. The exception is the luminal A subtype who tend to have a good prognosis regardless of obtaining a complete pCR. The unfavorable outcomes observed in the basal-like and HER2-enriched groups are attributable to those patients who did not achieve or attain a pCR with preoperative chemotherapy and therefore had a higher frequency of relapse or death (Carey et al. 2007; Fisher et al. 1998; Kuerer et al. 1999; Liedtke et al. 2008).

The treatment of the luminal A subgroup in the metastatic setting is often preferable to start with endocrine therapy consisting of the third-generation aromatase inhibitors (AI) in postmenopausal women, selective estrogen receptor modulators (SERMs) such as tamoxifen, and pure selective down-regulators of ER such as fulvestrant.

Luminal B breast cancer, despite expressing ER, is associated with increased risk of early relapse with endocrine therapy compared to the luminal A subtype. One explanation to explain this behavior is that luminal B breast cancer is associated with an increased expression of proliferation-related genes. Several biological pathways are identified as possible contributors to the poor outcomes, and novel agents targeting these pathways are being developed with the aim to improve survival. Some of these agents include inhibitors of insulin-like growth factor 1 receptor (IGF-1R), inhibitors of fibroblast growth factor receptor (FGFR), and inhibitors of mammalian target of rapamycin (mTOR).

The basal-like molecular subtype is correlated with an aggressive clinical course including an increased likelihood of disease recurrence and death (Dent et al. 2007). There are currently no specific targeted treatments for basal-like tumors due to the scarcity of data on which to base treatment decisions. The basal-like or triple-negative subtype of breast cancer represents an unmet therapeutic need and as such multiples therapeutic strategies are being investigated including DNA-damaging chemotherapy drugs such as platinum, inhibitors of poly (ADP-ribose) polymerase (PARP), and other novel agents.

The HER2 subtype carries a worse prognosis compared with other subtypes; however, the use of targeted anti-HER2 therapy, specifically adjuvant trastuzumab, a humanized monoclonal antibody directed against HER2, has improved survival in the HER2-overexpressing subtype of breast cancer. Five randomized trials of adjuvant trastuzumab showed a significant reduction of recurrence and mortality, as compared to no adjuvant trastuzumab (Viani et al. 2007). In addition, more recent clinical trials are focused on the development of newer agents that also block the HER2 receptor or downstream signaling, in addition to the combinations of newer HER2 targets which lead to dual HER2 blockade.

3   How Subtypes May Impact Prognosis?

There have been several analyses integrating molecular subtypes and their impact on prognosis. A pioneering study by Sorlie et al. noted a significant difference in overall survival between molecular subtypes (Sorlie et al. 2001, 2003) among patients with locally advanced breast cancer. The basal-like and HER2-enriched subtypes showed the poorest prognosis with both shorter time to progression and overall survival. The luminal subtypes are the most heterogeneous. However, the luminal A subtype had a considerably better prognosis compared with all other subtypes, and the luminal B subtype had an intermediate outcome.

Luminal A patients have a good prognosis with a relapse rate for early-stage luminal A breast cancer of 27.8 % being significantly lower than that for other subtypes (Kennecke et al. 2010). In addition, survival from the time of relapse is also longer (median 2.2 years).

Luminal B cancers have a worse prognosis than do luminal A cancers despite adjuvant systemic treatment. Cheang et al. (2009) analyzed tumors from patients with invasive breast carcinomas and found that luminal B breast cancer was statistically significantly associated with poor breast cancer recurrence-free and disease-specific survival in all adjuvant systemic treatment categories. For these reasons, treatment decisions regarding the luminal B subtype remain challenging.

HER2-positive tumors have been characterized by a poor prognosis, although in the last decade in which HER2-targeted therapies have been widely used, a substantial improvement in survival in both early-stage and metastatic HER2-positive breast cancer has been observed. Agents that target the HER2 receptor, heat shock protein inhibitors, anti-VEGF agents, and mTOR inhibitors are being studied in clinical trials and also provide alternative strategies for impacting HER2-driven disease, particularly following disease progression on an anti-HER2 therapy. There are many late-stage studies underway that will clarify the role of these newer therapies and the ways in which they will be integrated with established treatments.

Basal-like tumors have a worse prognosis compared with the luminal subtypes (Sorlie et al. 2003). They have a higher relapse rate in the first 3 years (Dent et al. 2007) despite having a high response to chemotherapy. They tend to have a high rate of p53 mutations, which may be an explanation for their poor prognosis and aggressive behavior. In addition, BRCA1 mutant tumors tend to be part of the basal-like subtype. BRCA1 is critical in DNA repair and its inactivation leads to the accumulation of errors and genetic instability favoring tumor growth. The BRCA pathway dysfunction can potentially be exploited therapeutically, e.g., inhibitors of the PARP enzyme and cross-linking agents as mentioned earlier. It is critical to continue to identify new therapeutic targets and design appropriate treatment strategies based on the biology of the distinct subtypes of breast cancer.

4   How Subtypes May Affect Patterns of Failure?

Evidence supporting the effect of molecular subtype on local and regional relapse has been demonstrated in a few studies. Nguyen et al. (2008) examined a cohort of 793 women with breast cancer treated with breast-conservation surgery. With 18 local events, the study found the HER2-enriched and basal-like subgroups were associated with an increased risk of local recurrence on multivariate analysis, 8.4 and 7.1 %, respectively. Local recurrence was low for the luminal A subtype (0.8 %) and the luminal B subtype 1.8 %. However, in this analysis, no patient received adjuvant trastuzumab. Haffty et al. (2006) observed a higher overall incidence of local recurrence in a cohort of 482 patients treated with breast-conservation surgery. They found the local recurrence rate to be 17 % at 5 years, with no difference noted between triple-negative and non-triple-negative breast cancer. There was a small, but not statistically significant, difference in nodal recurrence, with a higher risk observed in the triple-negative cancers versus the non-triple-negative cancer (5-year nodal recurrence rate of 6 % vs. 1 %, respectively, $p = 0.05$). Dent et al. (2009) also did not find a difference in local recurrence rates for basal-like breast cancer compared to other subtypes in a study of 1,601 patients.

Voduc et al. (2010) examined the risk of local and regional relapse in a large cohort of 2,985 patients with early-stage breast cancer. Luminal A tumors were associated with a low rate of local recurrence of 8 % at 10 years after either breast-conservation surgery or mastectomy, a result consistent across many studies, suggesting luminal A tumors exhibit the best overall prognosis (van't Veer et al. 2002). Since only 46 % of ER-positive patients in the Voduc study were treated with adjuvant tamoxifen, an even lower rate of relapse may be expected with the more consistent use of adjuvant hormonal therapy. Luminal A tumors also had infrequent regional relapse, 3 % at 10 years for both patients undergoing breast-conservation surgery and mastectomy.

Voduc et al. also found significant difference in local relapse rate in the HER2-enriched subgroup (21 % vs. 8 % for luminal A). The HER2 subtype was an independent marker for local recurrence after breast-conservation therapy. It is also important to note that with the widespread use of adjuvant trastuzumab, the risk of local recurrence would be expected to be lower. One may consider a radiation boost for some patients with other high-risk features to decrease the risk of local recurrence with this subtype.

Another important finding in the Voduc study was the high risk of locoregional relapse in luminal B tumors, identified using Ki-67. This study suggests luminal B is the second largest molecular subtype (35 % of hormone receptor-positive and HER2-negative tumors), and they were associated with significantly higher rates of local and regional relapse. Colleoni et al. (2004) found that high Ki-67 predicted for recurrence in small (<1 cm), node-negative breast cancers. Also, Mamounas et al. (2010) found that 25 % of a cohort of ER-positive, node-negative breast cancers had a high-risk recurrence score (Oncotype Dx), and this subgroup had a much higher risk of locoregional relapse compared with low-risk tumors (16 % vs. 4 %, respectively). These IHC markers can predict who may be at an increased risk of local and regional recurrence. Additional studies are required to identify the most effective treatment to address the higher risk of relapse seen with certain groups.

Preferential sites of distant metastatic disease have also been evaluated between the molecular subtypes. Sihto et al. (2011) analyzed 2,032 breast cancer core biopsies and found luminal A cancers had a propensity to give rise first to bone metastases, HER2-enriched cancers to liver and lung metastases, and basal-like cancers to liver and brain metastases. These findings are consistent with prior studies concluding biological subtypes are associated with site-specific distant recurrence.

5 Summary

Breast cancer is a heterogeneous disease with various clinical presentations, responses to treatment, and outcomes. While tumor size, histologic type, tumor grade, nodal involvement, and surgical margins affect prognosis, there are limitations on their prognostic value and there remains a great variation in breast cancers behavior. The molecular subtypes: (i) luminal A, (ii) luminal B, (iii) HER2-type, and (iv) basal-like have yielded insight into the heterogeneous biology and outcomes in patients with locally advanced disease. These subtypes have been found to be predictors of prognosis, response to systemic therapy, and locoregional recurrence.

References

Bertucci F, Finetti P et al (2005) Gene expression profiling identifies molecular subtypes of inflammatory breast cancer. Cancer Res 65:2170–2178

Carey LA, Dees EC et al (2007) The triple negative paradox: primary tumor chemosensitivity of breast cancer subtypes. Clin Cancer Res 13:2329–2334

Cheang MC, Chia SK et al (2009) Ki67 index, HER2 status, and prognosis of patients with luminal B breast cancer. J Natl Cancer Inst 101:736–750

Colleoni M, Rotmensz N et al (2004) Minimal and small size invasive breast cancer with no axillary lymph node involvement: the need for tailored adjuvant therapies. Ann Oncol 15:1633–1639

Colleoni M, Viale G et al (2008) Expression of ER, PGR, HER1, HER2, and response: a study of preoperative chemotherapy. Ann Oncol 19:465–472

Dent R et al (2007) Triple-negative breast cancer: clinical features and patterns of recurrence. Clin Cancer Res 13:4429–4434

Dent R, Hanna WM et al (2009) Pattern of metastatic spread in triple-negative breast cancer. Breast Cancer Res Treat 115:423–428

Fernandez-Morales LA, Segui MA et al (2007) Analysis of the pathologic response to primary chemotherapy in patients with locally advanced breast cancer grouped according to estrogen receptor, progesterone receptor, and HER2 status. Clin Breast Cancer 7:559–564

Fisher B, Bryant J et al (1998) Effect of preoperative chemotherapy on the outcome of women with operable breast cancer. J Clin Oncol 16:2672–2685

Gabos Z, Sinha R et al (2006) Prognostic significance of human epidermal growth factor receptor positivity for the development of brain metastasis after newly diagnosed breast cancer. J Clin Oncol 24(36):5658–5663

Goldstein NS, Decker D et al (2007) Molecular classification system identifies invasive breast carcinoma patients who are most likely and those who are least likely to achieve a complete pathologic response after neoadjuvant chemotherapy. Cancer 110:1687–1696

Guarneri V, Broglio K et al (2006) Prognostic value of pathologic complete response after primary chemotherapy in relation to hormone receptor status and other factors. J Clin Oncol 24:1037–1044

Haffty BG, Yang Q et al (2006) Locoregional relapse and distant metstasis in conservatively managed triple negative early-stage breast cancer. J Clin Oncol 24:5652–5657

Kennecke H, Yerushalmi R et al (2010) Metastatic behavior of breast cancer subtypes. J Clin Oncol 28(20):3271–3277

Kuerer HM, Newman LA et al (1999) Clinical course of breast cancer patients with complete pathologic primary tumor and axillary lymph node response to doxorubicin-based neoadjuvant chemotherapy. J Clin Oncol 17:460–469

Liedtke C, Mazouni C et al (2008) Response to neoadjuvant therapy and long-term survival in patients with triple-negative breast cancer. J Clin Oncol 26:1275–1281

Mamounas E, Tang G et al (2010) Association between the 21-gene recurrence score assay and risk of locoregional recurrence in node0negative, estrogen-receptor-positive breast cancer: results from NSABP B-14 and NSABP B-20. J Clin Oncol 28:1677–1683

Nguyen PL, Taghian AG et al (2008) Breast cancer subtype approximated by estrogen receptor, progesterone receptor, and HER2 is associated with local and distant recurrence after breast-conserving therapies. J Clin Oncol 26:2373–2378

Park S et al (2012) Characteristics and outcomes according to molecular subtypes of breast cancer as classified by a panel of four biomarkers using immunohistochemistry. Breast 21:50–57

Perou CM, Sorlie T et al (2000) Molecular portraits of human breast tumours. Nature 406:747–752

Rody A, Karn T et al (2007) The erb2+ cluster of the intrinsic gene set predicts tumor response of breast cancer patients receiving neoadjuvant chemotherapy with docetaxel, doxorubicin and cyclophosphamide within the GEPARTRIO trial. Breast 16:235–240

Rouzier R, Perou CM et al (2005) Breast cancer molecular subtypes respond differently to preoperative chemotherapy. Clin Cancer Res 11:5678–5685

Sanchez-Munoz A, Garcia-Tapiador AM et al (2008) Tumour molecular subtyping according to hormone receptors and HER2 status defines different pathological complete response to neoadjuvant chemotherapy in patients with locally advanced breast cancer. Clin Trans Oncol 10:646–653

Sihto H, Lundin J et al (2011) Breast cancer biological subtypes and protein expression predict for the preferential distant metastasis sites: a nationwide cohort study. Breast Cancer Res 13:R87

Sorlie T, Perou CM et al (2001) Gene expression patterns of breast carcinomas distinguish tumor subclasses with clinical implications. Proc Natl Acad Sci USA 98:10869–10874

Sorlie T, Tibshirani R et al (2003) Repeated observation of breast tumor subtypes in independent gene expression data sets. Proc Natl Acad Sci USA 100:8418–8423

Sotiriou C et al (2003) Breast cancer classification and prognosis based on gene expression profiles from a population-based study. Proc Natl Acad Sci USA 100:10393–10398

van't Veer LJ, Dai H et al (2002) Gene expression profiling predicts clinical outcome of breast cancer. Nature 415(6871):530–6

Viani G, Afonso S et al (2007) Adjuvant trastuzumab in the treatment of her-2 positive early breast cancer: a meta-analysis of published randomized trials. BMC Cancer 7:153

Voduc K, Cheang M et al (2010) Breast cancer subtypes and the risk of local and regional relapse. J Clin Oncol 28:1584–1691

Gene Amplification of ErbB-2: From Gene to Therapy

Kinnari Pandya and Clodia Osipo

Contents

K. Pandya · C. Osipo (✉)
Molecular Biology Program, Loyola University Chicago, Maywood, IL, USA
e-mail: cosipo@lumc.edu

C. Osipo
Department of Pathology/Oncology Institute, Loyola University Chicago, Maywood, IL, USA

C. Osipo
Department of Microbiology and Immunology, Loyola University Chicago, Maywood, IL, USA

Abstract

Breast cancer remains the second leading cause of cancer-related deaths worldwide. One of the main obstacles for finding a cure for breast cancer is the inherent heterogeneity of the disease. There are three main subtypes which include estrogen and/or progesterone (ER/PR)-positive, epidermal growth factor receptor-2 (ErbB-2/HER2)-positive, and triple negative that lack expression of ER or PR and express wild type levels of ErbB-2. The etiology of breast cancer development termed the tumorigenic process has been closely linked to gene amplification. Several genes have been shown to be amplified in breast cancer including the ErbB-2 gene on chromosome 17q12-21. The amplification of the ErbB-2 gene is a clear and defined indicator of ErbB-2-positive breast cancer development. In this chapter, we will review the classes of genes that are amplified and linked to breast cancer, discuss the significance of the ErbB-2 signaling pathway to breast cancer progression, targeted therapy, and drug resistance.

1 Gene Amplification: An Oncogenic Driver

Gene amplification refers to duplication of a chromosomal region that contains a gene. It occurs during uneven crossing-over during meiosis between disarranged homologous chromosomes. Multiple different biologically and clinically relevant genes are frequently duplicated or multiplied in breast cancer. Amplification of a gene is one way by which a gene can be overexpressed. The resulting overexpression of a proto-oncogene promotes uncontrolled cell proliferation and drives tumorigenesis by enabling constitutive activation of downstream signaling pathways and by inducing genetic instability, and thus, it usually predicts for poor prognosis. Some studies have shown a correlation between patient survival and number of gene amplifications. In addition, the function of genes involved plays a critical role in determining tumor characteristics. An early role for gene amplification in the development of breast cancer has been proposed. Gene amplification is a hallmark of malignant transformation and serves as a useful tool in determining targeted therapeutic options and/or prognosis.

The aim of this chapter was, therefore, to provide an overview of oncogenes that are amplified in breast cancer. Particularly, we will focus on understanding the role of ErbB-2 as an oncogenic driver and a therapeutic target in breast cancer.

2 Common Gene Amplifications in Breast Cancer

The following genes have been identified which, when amplified and overexpressed in breast cancer, are associated with high tumor grade, metastasis, poor prognosis, and decreased overall survival: *MYC* (48 %), *PRDM14* (34 %), *TOP2A* (32 %), *ADAM9* (32 %), *HER2* (28 %), *CCND1* (26 %), *EMSY* (25 %), *IKBKB* (21 %), *FGFR1* (17 %), *ESR1* (16 %), and *EGFR* (9 %). Frequently, the chromosomal regions that are amplified with high copy number during breast cancer development include 8p (*FGFR1, ADAM9, IKBKB*), 11q (*CCND1, EMSY*), and 17q (*PPARBP, HER2, TOP2A*). Most of the common amplifications in estrogen receptor-α (ERα)-positive breast tumors exhibit amplification of 8p and 11q chromosomal regions. However, amplification of the 17q chromosomal region has been identified in both ERα-positive and ERα-negative breast tumors.

Gene amplifications in breast cancer are frequent on chromosome 8p, 11q, and 17q, in which multiple driver oncogenes are amplified independently or together in various combinations. For example, tamoxifen-treated breast cancer patients often exhibit co-amplification of CCND1 and EMSY and this co-amplification predicts for poor survival. Both FGFR1 and CCND1 amplifications were associated with significantly reduced survival. In contrast, simultaneous amplification of HER2 and MYC has been shown to be associated with large tumors, reduced survival, and favorable outcome in response to trastuzumab, an anti-HER2 agent.

Amplification and co-amplification of several genes (oncogenes and tumor suppressors) have been shown to be involved in the development, maintenance, and progression of malignant breast cancer. However, the most comprehensive studies have been conducted in understanding the role of ErbB-2 (HER2/neu) as a proto-oncogene.

3 ErbB-2 Signaling Pathway (Fig. 1)

The human epidermal growth factor receptor-2 (ErbB-2, HER2/neu) is a type I transmembrane receptor tyrosine kinase. ErbB-2 and other family members (EGFR, ErbB-3, and ErbB-4) contain an N-terminal, extracellular ligand-binding domain, a transmembrane domain, and a C-terminal, intracellular tyrosine kinase domain. Unlike the other family members, ErbB-2 is considered to be an orphan receptor as it has no known ligand and ErbB-3 lacks tyrosine kinase activity. Under physiological conditions, ligand binding triggers hetero- or homo-dimerization of ErbB receptors resulting in auto- and transactivation of receptor kinase function. The active receptor tyrosine kinase then triggers various intracellular signaling pathways, including PI3'K and MAPK, resulting in cell survival and proliferation. Not all ErbB dimers exhibit equivalent signaling capacity; homo-dimers transmit weak signals compared to hetero-dimers. As ErbB-2 lacks a ligand, ErbB-2 hetero-dimerizes with other members of the ErbB family. However, the ErbB-2/ErbB-3 is considered the most potent hetero-dimer that promotes breast cancer cell proliferation and disease progression.

4 ErbB-2 Gene Amplification and Overexpression in Breast Cancer

The ErbB-2 proto-oncogene gene is amplified and is considered the main mechanism of ErbB-2 protein overexpression in 20–30 % of invasive breast cancers. ErbB-2-positive breast tumors have poor prognosis and are prone to early and frequent recurrence and metastases. Overexpression of ErbB-2 provides potent and constitutive activation of MAPK and PI3'K signaling pathways to drive breast tumorigenesis. Currently, trastuzumab (Herceptin®), a recombinant, humanized, monoclonal antibody, is a FDA-approved treatment for ErbB-2-amplified breast cancer. Trastuzumab specifically binds the juxta-membrane region of ErbB-2 at the cell surface to inhibit homo- or hetero-dimerization, thereby slowing growth by inhibiting activation and signaling. The best efficacy and positive therapeutic outcome with trastuzumab are observed in women with tumors that overexpress, have amplification, or have high activity of ErbB-2. Trastuzumab showed significant efficacy in the adjuvant settings with an overall response rate of 26 %, which increased to 80 % when combined with chemotherapeutic agents such as taxanes.

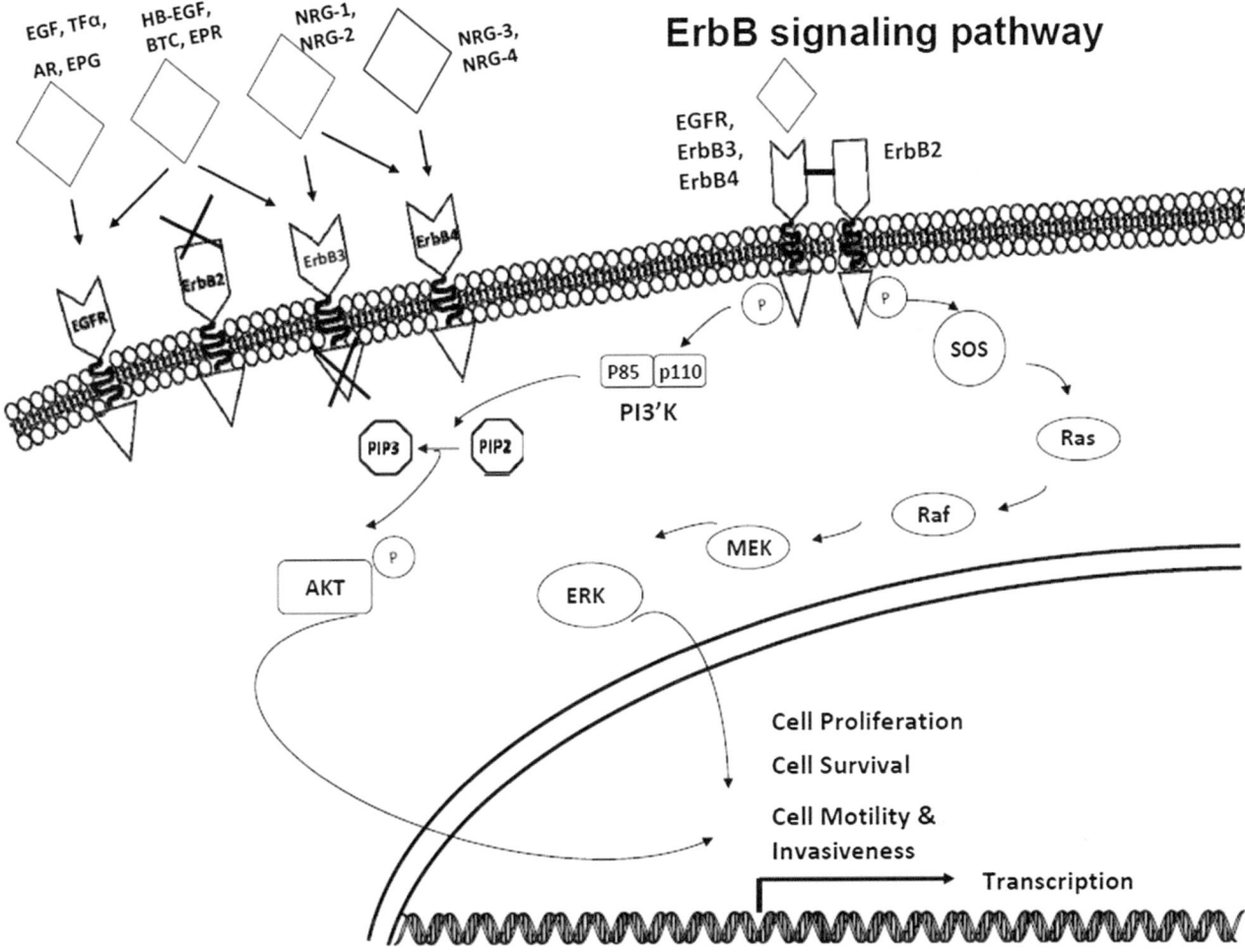

Fig. 1 ErbB signaling pathway

5 Mechanisms of Action (Fig. 2)

The exact mechanism by which trastuzumab inhibits ErbB-2 signaling is not yet fully understood. Some studies have suggested that trastuzumab binds to the extracellular domain of ErbB-2 and upon binding promotes internalization and degradation of ErbB-2 receptor. Other recent studies have demonstrated that trastuzumab selectively blocks ErbB-2/ErbB-3 hetero-dimerization. In addition, binding of trastuzumab to ErbB-2 blocks cleavage of the extracellular domain of the receptor, resulting in decreased levels of constitutively active and soluble p95-ErbB-2. As a result, trastuzumab acts as a potent anti-proliferative and anti-survival agent. Trastuzumab is also capable of inducing immune responses such as antibody-dependent cellular cytotoxicity (ADCC) against ErbB-2-overexpressing tumor cells. The Fc domain of trastuzumab engages with Fc receptors on immune effector cells (T cells) leading to lysis of tumor cells that overexpress ErbB-2. Furthermore, trastuzumab has anti-angiogenic effects. Trastuzumab initiates one important cellular response and that is cell cycle growth arrest in G1 phase, which is often accompanied by decrease in cyclin D1 levels and an increase in p27 levels. Trastuzumab induces little if any apoptosis.

6 Mechanisms of Resistance

Although trastuzumab has had a tremendous impact on improving survival for women with ErbB-2-positive breast cancer, trastuzumab resistance remains a major problem, particularly with metastatic tumors. Unfortunately, 66–88 % of women with metastatic breast cancer are resistant to trastuzumab as a single agent. Furthermore, many of the women who initially respond to trastuzumab-based treatments that include chemotherapy develop resistance within the first year of treatment. Approximately 15 % of women who receive trastuzumab will develop recurrent breast cancer, which almost always is metastatic to distant organs and ultimately results in death. In women with trastuzumab-resistant disease,

Mechanisms of Trastuzumab resistance

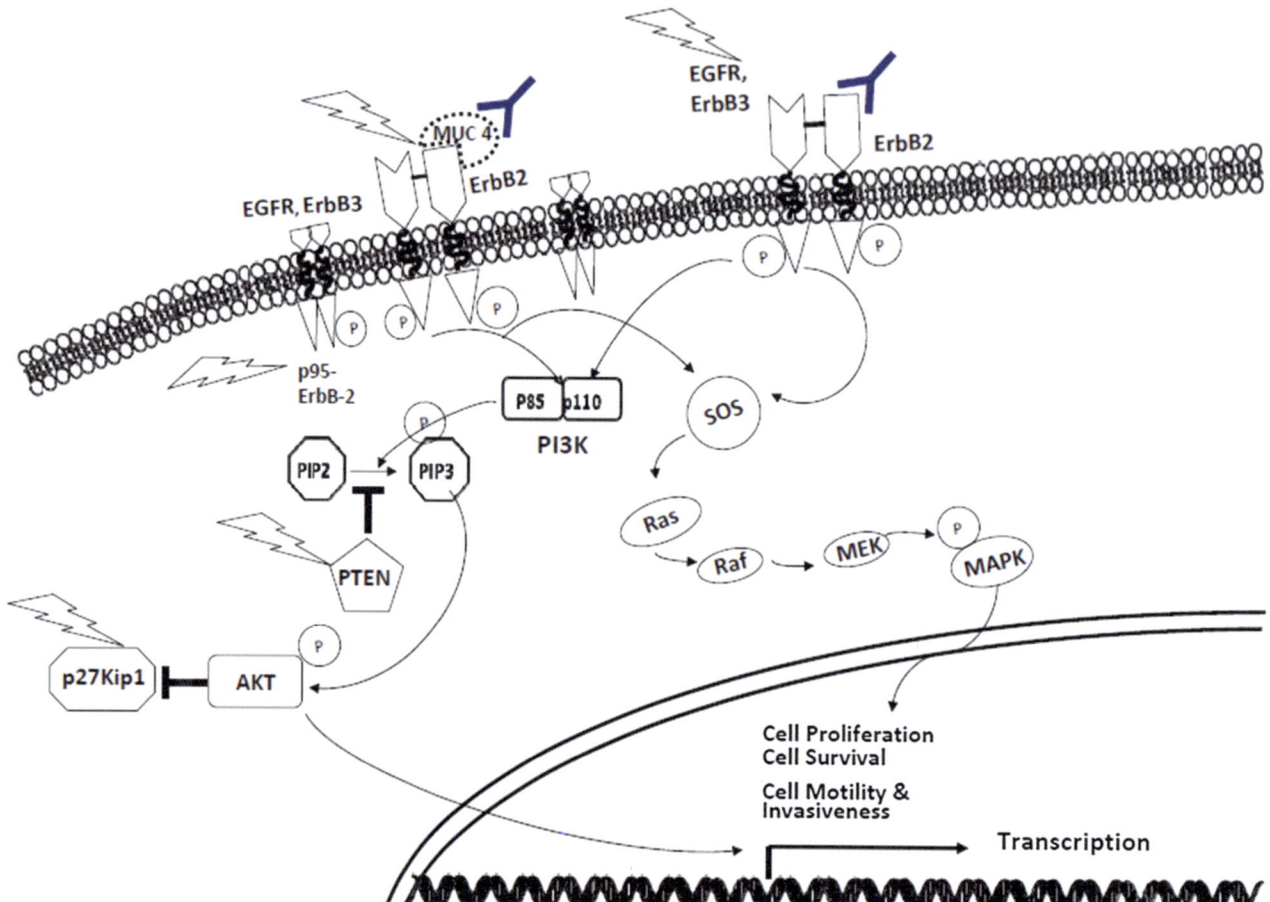

Fig. 2 Mechanisms of trastuzumab resistance

lapatinib, a small molecule, dual EGFR/ErbB-2 tyrosine kinase inhibitor (TKI), has been clinically proven to overcome some resistance to trastuzumab. However, resistance to lapatinib has been observed in patients within the first year of treatment. Thus, despite initial efficacy in the treatment of metastatic disease with anti-ErbB-2 agents, resistance occurs with no clinical means currently available to circumvent it. Thus, understanding the mechanisms responsible for resistance to ErbB-2-targeted therapies is critical to identify novel targets.

6.1 Functional Redundancy Among ErbB Family Members

ErbB family members are functionally redundant. The critical functions of ErbB signaling include dimerization, tyrosine phosphorylation, and activation of some redundant downstream signaling molecules. Even though trastuzumab inhibits ErbB-2 phosphorylation, it rarely blocks the dimerization of ErbB-2 with other ErbB family members. Recently,

long-term trastuzumab treatment of ErbB-2-positive breast cancer cells showed increase in EGFR and ErbB-3 expression. This indicates that alternate ErbB family dimers, such as ErbB-1/ErbB-1 and ErbB-1/ErbB-3 dimers, could possibly circumvent trastuzumab-induced blockade and promote growth and survival of breast tumors. Moreover, TGF-β has been shown to activate ErbB-3 in ErbB-2-overexpressing cells and subsequently the PI3'K pathway by enhancing phosphorylation and translocation of ADAM17 to the cell surface. This results in an increase in ErbB ligand shedding and desensitization of these cells to trastuzumab. Interestingly, from EGFR and ErbB-3 receptor knockdown studies, ErbB-3 has been shown to play a crucial role over EGFR in ErbB-2-amplified breast cancer. Therefore, a promising approach to treat trastuzumab resistance would be to design monoclonal antibodies that can be directed at dimerization of all the ErbB family members. Pertuzumab is a humanized, monoclonal antibody that was designed to specifically target hetero-dimers of the ErbB family. Recently, pertuzumab has shown significant efficacy when combined with trastuzumab in ErbB-2-positive metastatic breast cancer.

6.2 Role for Loss of Negative Regulators

Loss or decreased expression of negative regulators of signaling pathway activated by ErbB receptors has been implicated in resistance to trastuzumab. For example, the tumor suppressor phosphatase and tensin homolog (PTEN) is a negative regulator of the PI3'K/AKT signaling pathway. PTEN acts as a phosphatase to dephosphorylate PIP3 back to PIP2. This dephosphorylation results in inhibition of AKT pathway and subsequently controls cell survival, proliferation, and growth. ErbB-2-overexpressing breast tumors that express little to undetectable levels of PTEN respond poorly to trastuzumab therapy. Concurrently, constitutive PI3'K/ AKT kinase activity has also been shown to promote growth and proliferation of breast tumors. ErbB-2-overexpressing breast cancer cells that have heightened PI3'K/AKT signaling and reduced PTEN expression were shown to be the most sensitive to PI3'K or mTOR inhibitors. These inhibitors when combined with trastuzumab were able to overcome resistance both in vitro and in vivo breast tumor models. These results suggest that loss or low expression of PTEN and subsequent high AKT kinase activity induce trastuzumab resistance and serve as predictors of poor response to trastuzumab. Thus, inhibitors of the PI3'K/AKT/ mTOR signaling pathway need to be explored in combination with trastuzumab to prevent trastuzumab resistance. However, when tumor samples from trastuzumab-treated women were analyzed for PTEN and AKT status, the expression levels of PTEN and AKT did not significantly correlate with response to trastuzumab-based therapy, time to disease progression, or incidence of CNS metastases.

As described above, trastuzumab induces cell cycle growth arrest in G1 phase, which is often accompanied by an increase in a critical negative regulator of cell cycle progression, p27. Loss of expression of $p27^{Kip}$ has been implicated in trastuzumab resistance. The $p27^{Kip1}$ binds to cyclin E either alone or in a complex with cyclin-dependent kinase 2 (Cdk2) and inhibits the catalytic activity of Cdk2 to prevent Cdk2 from adding a phosphate group to its substrate. Trastuzumab induces a G1 cell cycle arrest within the breast tumor by enhancing the association of $p27^{Kip1}$ with cyclinE/ Cdk2 complexes, thus increasing the half-life of $p27^{Kip1}$ and preventing phosphorylation of $p27^{Kip1}$ by Cdk2 and subsequent ubiquitin-dependent degradation. Decreased $p27^{Kip1}$ levels and increased Cdk2 levels have been reported in trastuzumab-resistant breast cancer. Depletion of $p27^{Kip1}$ using either antisense or siRNA prevented trastuzumab-induced growth inhibition in ErbB-2-positive breast cancer cells. Conversely, overexpression of $p27^{Kip1}$ or preventing $p27^{Kip1}$ degradation using a proteasome inhibitor MG132 resensitized resistant cells to trastuzumab. These results suggest that $p27^{Kip1}$ could be yet another crucial marker of

trastuzumab resistance. However, $p27^{Kip1}$ protein expression has yet to predict response to trastuzumab-based therapy in patients with ErbB-2-overexpressing, metastatic breast cancer.

6.3 Accumulation of Soluble p95-ErbB-2

The efficacy of trastuzumab to inhibit ErbB-2 depends on its ability to recognize the juxta-membrane epitope of ErbB-2 and bind with high avidity. However, full-length ErbB-2 is a substrate for ADAM metalloproteinases and has been reported that a soluble form of ErbB-2 is detectable in serum of breast cancer patients. The remaining truncated version of ErbB-2 (p95) lacks the critical trastuzumab binding site within the extracellular domain. The p95-ErbB-2 can dimerize with other family members in a ligand-independent manner and constitutively turn on downstream signaling pathway. Approximately 30 % of ErbB-2-amplified breast cancers exhibit p95-ErbB-2 expression and is associated with adverse outcome and resistance to trastuzumab. Breast cancer cell lines (expressing low levels of ErbB-2) transfected with p95-ErbB-2 showed sensitivity only to lapatinib, whereas transfection with full-length ErbB-2 exhibited sensitivity to both trastuzumab and lapatinib. A retrospective analysis of 46 patients confirmed that expression of p95-ErbB-2 increased tumor growth and led to trastuzumab resistance, whereas expression of wild-type ErbB-2 maintained sensitivity to trastuzumab. These data suggest that tumors expressing constitutively active p95-ErbB-2 maintain their dependence on ErbB-2 activity for proliferation and may respond better to alternative approaches to inhibiting ErbB-2.

6.4 Role for MUC4: Altered Receptor– Antibody Interaction

Trastuzumab exerts its anti-tumor activity by binding and inhibiting ErbB-2 at the cell surface. Thus, altering the interaction between ErbB-2 and trastuzumab could serve as an emerging mechanism that could contribute to trastuzumab resistance. For example, MUC4, a membrane-associated mucin, functions by modulating ErbB-2 signaling. The ascites sialoglycoprotein-2 (ASGP-2) subunit of glycoprotein MUC4 directly interacts with ErbB-2 via an EGF-like domain, masking ErbB-2 and inhibiting trastuzumab binding to ErbB-2. Elevated MUC4 expression is observed during acquired trastuzumab resistance. This interaction was associated with increase in phosphorylation of ErbB-2 at tyrosine 1248, which plays a major role in ErbB-2-driven tumorigenesis. MUC4 activates ErbB-2, without affecting the expression of ErbB-2. Inhibition of MUC4 using siRNA increased trastuzumab binding and sensitized resistant breast cancer cells to trastuzumab. Thus, novel agents targeting MUC4 expression and/or function in combination with trastuzumab might prove to be advantageous in the treatment of resistant tumors.

6.5 Crosstalk Between ErbB-2 and Notch Signaling Pathways

Recently, Notch signaling has emerged as a target for the treatment of breast cancer. Notch-1 is another breast oncogene and a potent cell fate receptor. Women diagnosed with breast cancer that co-overexpress Notch-1 and its ligand Jagged-1 have the poorest overall survival. Notch-1 and Notch-4 are breast oncogenes that promote breast cancer tumorigenesis by simultaneously inhibiting differentiation, promoting survival, and proliferation. We have identified, Notch-1, as a novel target in trastuzumab-resistant breast cancer. Based on our recent findings, we showed that ErbB-2 inhibits Notch-1 activity. We showed that when breast cancer cells that overexpress ErbB-2 are treated with trastuzumab, the unintended consequence is activation of Notch-1. This increased Notch-1 signaling decreased the effectiveness of trastuzumab. We recently showed using preclinical xenograft models that simultaneous inhibition of Notch and ErbB-2 significantly decreased recurrence of ErbB-2-positive breast tumors and reversed trastuzumab resistance.

7 Alternative Treatment Options for ErbB-2-Overexpressing Breast Cancer

Despite the advances that have been made by trastuzumab and lapatinib, patients with metastatic breast cancer develop resistance to anti-ErbB-2 agents during the course of treatment and eventually develop disease progression. The table below shows alternative treatment strategies for patients with resistant breast cancer.

ErbB-2 dimerization inhibitor	Pertuzumab
ErbB-2 ADCC	T-DM1
PI3'K inhibitor	LY294002
Tyrosine kinase inhibitors	Lapatinib, neratinib, BIBW 2992
mTOR inhibitors	Everolimus
HSP90 inhibitors	Tanespimycin
VEGF receptor inhibitors	Bevacizumab
IGF-1R inhibitors	NVP-AEW541, CP-751871
Notch pathway inhibitors	GSI

8 Conclusions

Overexpression of ErbB-2 as a result of gene amplification has provided an outstanding opportunity to develop targeted therapy for breast cancer. It has for the most part been a very successful example of how identification of oncogene amplification has led to an FDA-approved treatment strategy. Trastuzumab has had a tremendous impact on improving survival for women with ErbB-2-positive breast cancer. However, resistance to trastuzumab remains a major problem, particularly among women with metastatic disease. Thus, elucidating the molecular mechanisms underlying intrinsic or acquired anti-ErbB-2 drug resistance may provide crucial information about patients that fail to respond to therapy or develop resistance within the first year of their treatment. Thus, there is an immediate urge for genomic, transcriptomic, and proteomic approaches to better understand the mechanisms of ErbB-2-targeted drug resistance. Some of the molecular mechanisms for acquired resistance and possibly intrinsic resistance summarized in this book chapter include overexpression of redundant ErbB family members, overexpression of MUC4, and loss of negative regulators (PTEN and p27^{Kip1}). We have identified a novel biomarker of trastuzumab resistance: Notch-1. Compensatory increase in Notch-1 activity upon trastuzumab treatment could provide a survival advantage to breast cancer cells, driving tumorigenesis, and resistance. Activated Notch-1 may contribute to resistance by regulating previously identified molecular markers of trastuzumab resistance, activating alternative signaling pathways, and potentiating crosstalk between the tumor and its surrounding microenvironment. Thus, a thorough analysis of the role of Notch signaling in ErbB-2-amplified breast cancers would provide an evidential rationale of whether targeting the Notch pathway could improve the way trastuzumab-resistant ErbB-2-positive breast cancer patients are treated today.

Further Reading

Gajria D, Chandarlapaty S (2011) HER2-amplified breast cancer: mechanisms of trastuzumab resistance and novel targeted therapies. Expert Rev Anticancer Ther 2:263–275

Mehta K, Osipo C (2009) Trastuzumab resistance: role for notch signaling. Sci World J 9:1438–1448

Moelans CB, de Weger RA, Monsuur HN, Vijzelaar R, van Diest PJ (2010) Molecular profiling of invasive breast cancer by multiplex ligation-dependent probe amplification-based copy number analysis of tumor suppressor and oncogenes. Mod pathol 7:1029–1039

Mukohara T (2011) Mechanisms of resistance to anti-human epidermal growth factor receptor 2 agents in breast cancer. Cancer Sci 1:1–8

Osipo C, Patel P, Rizzo P, Clementz AG, Hao L, Golde TE, Miele L (2008) ErbB-2 inhibition activates Notch-1 and sensitizes breast cancer cells to a gamma-secretase inhibitor. Oncogene 37:5019–5032

Pandya K, Meeke K, Clementz AG, Rogowski A, Roberts J, Miele L, Albain KS, Osipo C (2011) Targeting both Notch and ErbB-2 signalling pathways is required for prevention of ErbB-2-positive breast tumour recurrence. Br J Cancer 6:796–806

Slamon D, Pegram M (2001) Rationale for trastuzumab (Herceptin) in adjuvant breast cancer trials. Semin Oncol 28:13–19

Slamon DJ, Godolphin W, Jones LA, Holt JA, Wong SG, Keith DE, Levin WJ, Stuart SG, Udove J, Ullrich A, Press MF (1989) Studies of the HER-2/neu proto-oncogene in human breast and ovarian cancer. Science 244:707–712

Current Clinical Role of Genetic Profiling in Breast Cancer

Ruta Rao, Mashrafi Ahmed, and William T. Leslie

Contents

Abstract

Genetic profiling of breast cancer is emerging as an important prognostic and predictive tool, especially for patients with early-stage breast cancer. Several genetic profile assays are already commercially available, and others are being developed and tested. OncotypeDx, a 21-gene assay, and MammaPrint, a 70-gene assay are the most extensively evaluated tests. Currently, three prospective trials to assess the predictive value of gene signature assays in certain subgroups of breast cancer are ongoing. These are the Trial Assigning Individualized Options for Treatment (Rx) (TAILORx) trial, the endocrine-responsive breast cancer (RxPONDER) trial for 21-gene recurrence score and Microarray In Node-negative Disease may Avoid ChemoTherapy (MINDACT) trial using the 70-gene signature.

1   Introduction

Recent research has shown that breast cancer is a heterogeneous disease at the genetic level. The variations in gene expression affect the clinical behavior and course of the disease. In one of the initial studies, Perou and colleagues analyzed the gene expression patterns of 65 breast cancer specimens from 42 individuals (Perou et al. 2000). They found that the tumors showed a wide variation in the patterns of gene expression. However, the patterns from two tumor samples from the same individual were more similar to each other than to any other sample. Based on their findings, they were able to identify what are now known as the biological subtypes of breast cancer: estrogen receptor (ER)-positive, luminal A and B, basal-like, Erb-B2+, normal, and claudin-low. These subtypes of breast cancer have different natural histories and survival patterns, as well as different patterns of response to therapy. Gene expression profiling is not yet routinely performed in the analysis of a breast tumor, so identification of these subtypes is not currently being utilized

R. Rao (✉) · W.T. Leslie
Rush University Medical Center, 1653 W Congress Pkwy,
Chicago, IL 60612, USA
e-mail: ruta_d_rao@rush.edu

M. Ahmed
Saint Joseph Hospital, 2900 N Lake Shore Dr, Chicago,
IL 60657, United States

J. Strauss et al. (eds.), *Breast Cancer Biology for the Radiation Oncologist*, Medical Radiology. Radiation Oncology,
DOI: 10.1007/174_2014_1044, © Springer-Verlag Berlin Heidelberg 2014
Published Online: 6 December 2014

clinically. Instead, tumors are now classified clinically based on their ER, progesterone receptor (PR), and human epidermal growth factor receptor-2 (HER2) status. For practical purposes, the subtypes can be approximated using this clinical data, although there is no perfect correlation between the results of gene expression array tests.

Over the last two decades, significant improvements have been made in breast cancer mortality rates. The 5-year relative survival rate for women with breast cancer increased from 63 % in the early 1960s to 90 % today (American Cancer Society 2011). This improvement has likely been due to earlier diagnosis and improvements in therapy, among other reasons. Adjuvant therapy has been shown to significantly improve disease-free and overall survival in both premenopausal and postmenopausal patients up to 70 years of age with node-negative or node-positive breast cancer. Given the multitude of currently available medical treatments for breast cancer, it is a challenge to select the appropriate adjuvant therapy for an individual patient. Genomic assays have recently become powerful tools in predicting recurrence and mortality, which allows the refinement of therapeutic approaches.

Unlike conventional clinical prognostic factors, genetic profiling has not been validated in prospective randomized clinical trials. Though the results of these tests are reproducible, they are expensive and have limited availability. Also, there is a paucity of data comparing the available tests. Nevertheless, they have the potential to improve and individualize clinical decision making. Until now, decisions regarding adjuvant chemotherapy have been determined by factors including age, performance status, tumor size, tumor grade, tumor stage, lymph node involvement, and ER, PR, and HER2 status. These factors are combined in guidelines such as the National Institutes of Health (NIH) Consensus Development criteria (National Institutes of Health 2000; (Eifel et al. 2001), the St. Gallen expert opinion criteria (Goldhirsch et al. 2001, 2005), the National Comprehensive Cancer Network Guidelines (2011), and a Web-based algorithm, Adjuvant! Online (Ravdin et al. 2001; Adjuvant Inc. 2012). These guidelines suggest that the majority of women with node-negative, estrogen receptor-positive breast cancer should be offered chemotherapy. However, this approach will likely result in overtreatment in many women since only a minority of these patients will develop recurrent disease (Eifel et al. 2001; NCCN 2011). It is generally thought that patients with poor prognostic features benefit the most from adjuvant therapy. For example, axillary nodal involvement has been considered one of the most important prognostic features, with an increasing number of axillary nodes correlating with a more unfavorable clinical outcome (Carter et al. 1989; Page 1991; Rosen et al. 1989). It is thought that patients with positive nodes are most likely to benefit from adjuvant chemotherapy, with an absolute benefit of 6–15 % at 5 years (Early Breast Cancer Trialists' Collaborative Group 2005). However, this population benefit is not true for all individuals, since 25–30 % of node-positive patients will remain free of distant metastases even without systemic adjuvant therapy (Joensuu et al. 1998). Therefore, recommending adjuvant chemotherapy based on the nodal status alone results in overtreatment of a significant portion of patients. If more reliable tests could identify which high-risk patients would benefit from adjuvant chemotherapy, many other patients could be spared from the unnecessary toxicities.

This chapter will focus on the different types of gene expression profiling tests that are available for clinical use in breast cancer and on new tests that are still being developed.

2   Gene Expression Profiling

The level of gene expression reflects the activity of a particular gene. The transcription of genetic DNA into messenger RNA (mRNA) is the first step in gene expression. Technologies such as DNA microarray analysis and real-time reverse-transcriptase polymerase chain reaction (RT-PCR) allow the simultaneous measurement of multiple gene transcriptions. The two FDA-approved tests that are now available in the clinical setting are the 21-gene RT-PCR assay (Oncotype Dx) and the 70-gene signature (MammaPrint). Others that will be described are a two-gene signature (HOX13:IL17BR ratio), Mammostrat, the Rotterdam 76-gene signature, 11-gene EP score, 97-gene genomic grade index, Breast Cancer Index, and the wound-response gene expression.

3   21 Gene RT-PCR Assay (Oncotype DX)

Oncotype DX is a 21-gene assay that measures the expression of 16 tumor-related and 5 reference genes by RT-PCR (reverse-transcriptase polymerase chain reaction). It can be performed on formalin-fixed, paraffin-embedded tissue samples. The 16 tumor-related genes were prospectively chosen from a 250-candidate gene set, selected from an extensive literature review and analyzed for expression and relation to relapse-free survival (RFS) across 3 independent studies of 447 patients, which demonstrated a consistent statistical link between these genes and distant breast cancer recurrence (Paik et al. 2003; Cobleigh et al. 2005; Esteban et al. 2003). Five of the genes are in the proliferation group (Ki-67, STK15, Survivin, Cyclin B1, and MYBL2), two in the HER2 group (HER2 and GRB7), four in the estrogen receptor group (ER, PR, Bcl2, and Scube2), two in the invasion group (Stromelysin3 and Cathepsin L2), and 3 unaligned (macrophage marker CD68, anti-apoptosis gene BAG1, GSTM1). Some of the genes were already well described in the breast cancer literature, while others were relatively new. Based on these 21 genes, an algorithm was developed to determine a RS, which is divided into low-risk (<18), intermediate-risk (18–30), and high-risk (≥31) categories (Fig. 1).

The 21-gene RT-PCR assay has both prognostic and predictive values. It estimates the likelihood of disease recurrence within 10 years, and it predicts the benefit of chemotherapy and tamoxifen in reducing the risk of recurrence. The use of this test is endorsed by the American Society of Clinical Oncology for women with ER-positive, lymph node-negative, early-stage breast cancer (Harris et al. 2007), the NCCN guidelines 2011, and the St. Gallen International Expert Consensus (Goldhirsch et al. 2009). According to the NCCN guidelines, the 21-gene RT-PCR assay should be considered in determining the need for adjuvant chemotherapy for patients with hormone receptor-positive, HER2-negative tumors that are pT1b-pT3 and N0 or N1mi (≤2 mm axillary nodal metastases). If the RS is low risk (<18), adjuvant endocrine therapy alone is recommended. If the RS is intermediate risk (18–31), chemotherapy should be considered, and if it is high risk (≥31), chemotherapy is recommended.

The 21-gene RT-PCR assay was retrospectively validated in the National Surgical Adjuvant Breast and Bowel Project Trial (NSABP) B-14 (Paik et al. 2004). The original trial prospectively randomized 2,828 node-negative, ER-positive women to receive tamoxifen or placebo, and an additional 1,235 patients were registered to tamoxifen in the 10-month period following closure of the trial in 1988, resulting in a total of 2,617 eligible tamoxifen-treated patients (Fisher et al. 1996, 1999, 2001a, b). RT-PCR was successfully performed in 668 of 675 available tumor blocks. Fifty-one percent of the patients were classified as low risk, 22 % were intermediate risk, and 27 % were high risk. One primary objective was to determine whether the proportion of patients who were free of disease for more than 10 years was significantly greater in the low-risk group than in the high-risk group. The 10-year disease-free survival was 93.2 % for patients in the low-risk group as compared to 69.5 % in the high-risk group, $p < 0.001$. The RS also provided significant predictive power that was independent of age and tumor size in a multivariate analysis ($p < 0.001$) (Fig. 2 and Table 1).

The 21-gene RT-PCR assay was further validated in a large population-based, case–controlled study of node-negative, ER-positive patients who were not treated with adjuvant chemotherapy (Habel et al. 2006). Of 4,694 patients diagnosed with invasive breast cancer between 1985 and 1994, a blinded analysis was performed on the tissue of 220 women who had died from breast cancer and 570 women who had not. The RS correlated with the risk of breast cancer

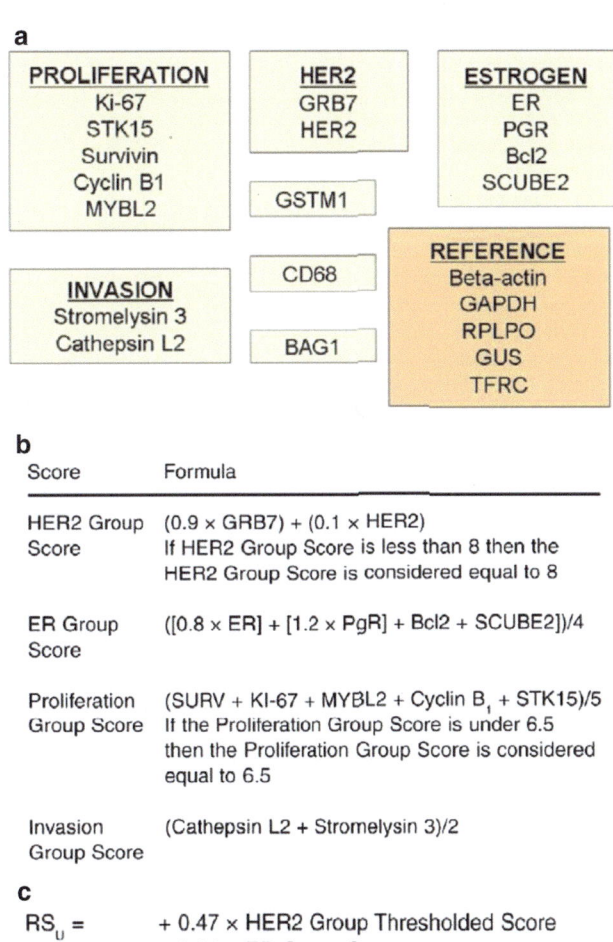

Fig. 1 **a** The final gene list (16 cancer-related and five reference genes) and summary score (recurrence score) algorithm for this assay were developed by analyzing the results of three independent preliminary breast cancer studies (training sets) with a total of 447 patients. The recurrence score, on a scale from 0 to 100, is derived from the reference-normalized expression measurements in four steps. In the first step, the expression for each gene is normalized relative to the expression of the five reference genes (b-actin, GAPDH, GUS, RPLPO, and TFRC). Reference-normalized expression measurements range from 0 to 15, where a 1-unit increase reflects approximately a twofold increase in RNA. **b** In the second step, the HER2 group score, the ER group score, the proliferation group score, and the invasion group score are calculated from individual gene expression measurements. **c** In the third step, the recurrence score unscaled (RSu) is calculated using coefficients that were predefined based on regression analysis of gene expression and recurrence in the three training studies (providence, rush, and NSABP B-20). A plus sign indicates that increased expression is associated with recurrence risk. A minus sign indicates that increased expression is associated with decreased recurrence risk. *Source* Habel et al. 2006

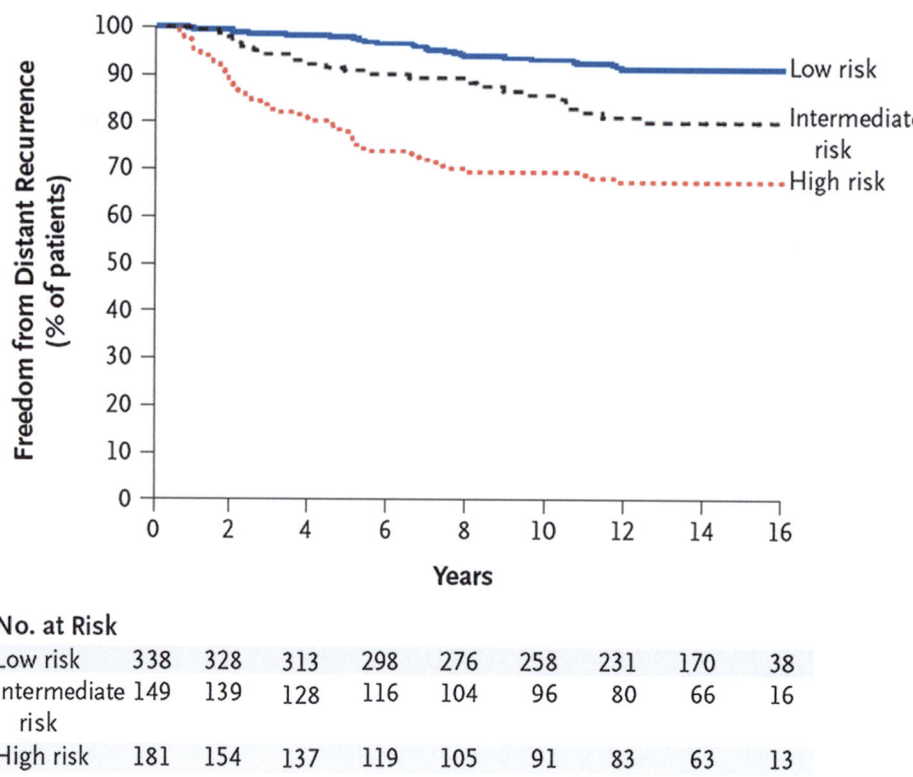

Fig. 2 Likelihood of distance recurrence, according to recurrence score categories. A low risk was defined as a recurrence score of less than 18, an intermediate risk as a score of 18 or higher but less than 31, and a high risk as a score of 31 or higher. There were 28 recurrences in the low-risk groups, 25 in the intermediate-risk group, and 56 in the high-risk group. The difference between the groups is significant (P <0.001). *Source* Paik et al. 2004

No. at Risk

Low risk	338	328	313	298	276	258	231	170	38
Intermediate risk	149	139	128	116	104	96	80	66	16
High risk	181	154	137	119	105	91	83	63	13

Table 1 Kaplan–Meier estimates of the rate of distant recurrence at 10 years, according to recurrence score-risk categories

Risk category	Percentage of patients	Rate of distant recurrence at 10 yr (95 % confidence interval) (%)
Low	51	6.8 (4.0–9.6)
Intermediate	22	14.3 (8.3–20.3)
High	27	30.5 (23.6–37.4)*

*$P < 0.001$ for the comparison with the low-risk category (*Source* Paik et al. 2004)

death in this population, after adjusting for tumor size and grade, in both tamoxifen-treated and tamoxifen-untreated patients ($P = 0.003$ and $P = 0.03$, respectively). The RS provided information independent of tumor size and grade. The relative risk estimations for RS in the ER-positive patients were similar to those in NSABP B-14 (Paik et al. 2004).

In a single smaller analysis, the 21-gene RT-PCR assay did not correlate with recurrence-free survival (Esteva et al. 2005). The RS was performed on archival paraffin-embedded tissue samples of 144 patients with node-negative, invasive breast cancer who received no systemic adjuvant therapy. The RS was not predictive of distant disease recurrence. There was a high concordance between the RT-PCR results and immunohistochemical assays for estrogen receptor, progesterone receptor, and human epidermal growth factor receptor 2 status. When attempting to reconcile the results of this series to others, it is important to note

that in this series alone, ER-negative patients were included. In addition, a high tumor grade was associated with a better prognosis in this study, calling into question the validity of this series.

In addition to its prognostic value, the 21-gene RT-PCR assay has been shown to be predictive of benefit from tamoxifen and chemotherapy. In NSABP B-14, patients treated with tamoxifen were compared to those treated with placebo. The patients with the low- and intermediate-risk RS who received tamoxifen had large improvements in disease-free survival, while those with high-risk RS had a smaller benefit (Paik et al. 2004). NSABP B-20 was a phase III trial that randomized 2,363 patients to receive tamoxifen either alone or tamoxifen with chemotherapy (either cyclophosphamide, methotrexate, and fluorouracil or methotrexate and fluorouracil) (Paik et al. 2006). RT-PCR was successfully performed in 651 patients (227 randomized to tamoxifen, 424 randomized to tamoxifen plus chemotherapy). The distribution of age, tumor size, tumor grade, and hormone receptor status was similar to the entire trial population. In this group, 54.2 % of the patients were low-risk, 20.6 % intermediate-risk, and 25.2 % high-risk RS. For the low-risk patients, the addition of chemotherapy added no benefit in reducing the risk of distant recurrence at 10 years (relative risk, 1.31; 95 % CI, 0.46–3.78; increase of 1.1 % in absolute risk), while there was a large reduction in distant recurrence at 10 years for the high-risk category (relative risk, 0.26; 95 % CI, 0.13–0.53; decrease of 27.6 % in absolute risk).

The benefit from chemotherapy was less clear for patients in the intermediate-risk group (relative risk, 0.61; 95 % CI, 0.24–1.59; 1.8 % increase in absolute risk). Given the uncertainty in the estimate, a clinically important benefit could not be excluded for the intermediate-risk patients.

The value of the RS in predicting response to neoadjuvant chemotherapy in locally advanced breast cancer has been confirmed in two studies. In one study, 89 patients were treated with neoadjuvant doxorubicin and paclitaxel, and 11 (12 %) had a complete pathologic response (pCR) (Gianni et al. 2005). The RS was positively associated with the likelihood of pCR ($p = 0.005$), suggesting that patients who had the greatest risk of distant recurrence are likely to derive the greatest benefit from chemotherapy. In the second study, 97 patients had core biopsies taken prior to treatment with neoadjuvant docetaxel (Chang et al. 2008). Eighty (82 %) of the specimens had sufficient RNA for RT-PCR, and in 72 (74 %) of the patients, clinical response data were available. Clinical complete responses were more likely in the high-RS group ($p = 0.008$). Tumors with significant increases in the proliferative gene group and decreases in the ER gene group were most likely to respond to chemotherapy.

The 21-gene RT-PCR assay was evaluated in a more contemporary population of women with early-stage, hormone receptor-positive, node-negative and node-positive, operable breast cancer in an analysis of the Arimidex, Tamoxifen, Alone or in Combination (ATAC) trial (Dowsett et al. 2010). In this trial, postmenopausal women were randomized to anastrozole, tamoxifen, or both drugs. Among the 4,160 patients in the monotherapy arms, there were 1,231 evaluable patients in whom the RS was determined; 71 % were node-negative, 25 % were node-positive, and 4 % had unknown nodal status. In both node-negative and node-positive patients, the RS was significantly associated with time to distant recurrence by multivariate analyses ($p < 0.001$ and $p = 0.002$, respectively). The RS also showed significant prognostic value beyond that provided by adjuvant! online ($p < 0.001$). In node-negative patients, 9-year distant recurrence (DR) rates in low (RS < 18), intermediate (RS 18–30), and high-RS (RS ≥ 31) groups were 4, 12, and 25 %, respectively, and 17, 28, and 49 %, respectively, in node-positive patients. This study validated the RS in the tamoxifen-treated population. In this analysis, the relative risk reduction was similar across the different RS groups. Overall, the ATAC trial demonstrated a 16 % relative reduction in the rate of distant recurrence for patients treated with anastrozole. This analysis established that the relationship between the RS and DR could be applied to patients treated with anastrozole, with an approximate 16 % adjustment for the lower risk of distant recurrence for those patients. Also, this study confirmed the poor correlation between the RS and adjuvant! online although both measures provided substantial independent prognostic information.

The 21-gene RT-PCR assay is currently recommended for use in women with node-negative, hormone receptor-positive tumors, although some of the original work was done in node-positive patients (Cobleigh et al. 2005). In one study, RNA was extracted from 78 paraffin tumor blocks of patients with breast cancer diagnosed between 1979 and 1999. All of the patients had ten or more lymph nodes involved (median 15 lymph nodes). At the time of publication, 77 % of the patients had distant disease recurrence or breast cancer-related death. When the RS was obtained, 11 patients (14 %) had a RS < 18 with a rate of distant recurrence at 10 years of 29 %, 19 patients (24 %) had a RS of 18–31 with a rate of distant recurrence at 10 years of 72 %, and 48 patients (62 %) had a RS of ≥ 31 with a rate of distant recurrence at 10 years of 80 %. This showed that there was a subset of node-positive patients with a low RS who had a prolonged disease-free survival.

Recently, the RS has been tested retrospectively in a randomized trial of node-positive women, Southwest Oncology Group (SWOG) 8814 (Albain et al. 2010). The original trial showed that chemotherapy with CAF (cyclophosphamide, doxorubicin and 5-fluorouracil) given before tamoxifen improved disease-free and overall survival when compared to tamoxifen alone in postmenopausal women with node-positive, ER-positive breast cancer. The two primary objectives of the retrospective analysis were to determine whether the RS assay could provide prognostic information for women with node-positive disease treated with tamoxifen alone and whether the assay could identify a subset of node-positive patients who did not benefit from the addition of chemotherapy. An analysis was performed on 367 specimens from the original trial (40 % of the patients in the CAF-T and T-alone groups). This subset of patients resembled the patients in the original study except for a slightly lower number of positive lymph nodes and smaller tumor size. When adjusted for the number of positive lymph nodes, the benefit in disease-free and overall survival was similar for CAF-T over T alone, as was seen in the parent trial. The RS was highly prognostic in the T-alone group, with 10-year DFS estimates of 60, 49, and 43 % for low-, intermediate-, and high-risk categories. The RS was also a strong predictive factor of benefit from CAF chemotherapy. There was no benefit for chemotherapy in women who had a low-risk RS (stratified log-rank $p = 0.97$; HR 1.02, 95 % CI 0.54–1.93), whereas those with a high-risk RS had a significant improvement in disease-free survival (stratified log-rank $p = 0.033$; HR 0.59, 0.35–1.01). This analysis suggests that there may be subsets of women with ER-positive, node-positive disease who do not derive additional benefit from adjuvant anthracycline-based chemotherapy.

The 21-gene RT-PCR assay has been shown to be superior to standard clinical and pathologic factors (Goldstein et al. 2008). In a study of 465 patients with hormone receptor-positive breast cancer with zero to three positive axillary nodes, the RS was a powerful prognostic factor for recurrence in both node-negative and node-positive disease ($p < 0.001$ for both). It was more strongly associated with recurrence than clinical variables, which were integrated by an algorithm modeled after adjuvant! that was adjusted to 5-year outcomes. The 5-year recurrence rate was only 5 % or less for the estimated 46 % of patients who have a low RS (<18).

The prognostic utility of the RS and adjuvant! was compared in the 668 tamoxifen-treated patients in NSABP B-14, 227 tamoxifen-treated patients in NSABP B-20 and 424 chemotherapy and tamoxifen-treated patients in NSABP B-20 (Tang et al. 2011). Adjuvant! uses patient and tumor characteristics to predict the clinical outcome, and is routinely used in practice (Ravdin et al. 2001; Olivotto et al. 2005). Adjuvant! also utilizes the results of the Early Breast Cancer Clinical Trialists' Collaborative Group (EBCTCG) overview to assign benefit from adjuvant therapies, assuming the same proportional reduction in recurrence and mortality across different prognostic categories (EBCTCG 2005). The results showed that the RS and adjuvant! were independently prognostic for the risk of distant recurrence. In the NSABP B-20 cohort with RS results available, the RS was significantly predictive of chemotherapy benefit (interaction $p = 0.031$ for DRFI, $p = 0.011$ for OS), whereas adjuvant! was not significantly predictive (interaction $p = 0.99$ and $p = 0.311$, respectively).

The 21-gene RT-PCR can reclassify patients who were considered high risk by conventional prognostic markers to a low-risk group. Paik et al. (2005) showed that the 21-gene RT-PCR assay was more accurately predictive than the St. Gallen or National Comprehensive Cancer Network risk stratification guidelines, and this could be used to change some patient decisions about chemotherapy. In this study, about half of the patients who were in the high-risk category as defined by the NCCN guidelines could be reclassified as low-risk by the 21-gene RT-PCR assay, with a 10-year relapse risk of 7 % (CI, 4–11 %). This is similar to the relapse rate seen in the low-risk RS group without the NCCN information. A separate study also compared RS with adjuvant! In the 668 tamoxifen-treated patients from NSABP-B14 (Bryant 2005), 32 % of the patients were low-risk according to both algorithms. Overall, there is about a 48 % concordance between the RS and adjuvant! online-risk categories. About 18 % of patients are classified as low risk according to one algorithm, but high risk according to the other. The RS correlated more strongly with outcome than did adjuvant! These findings suggest that the greatest impact of the RS is in reclassifying patients from high to low risk, thereby reducing the number of women who would be given chemotherapy unnecessarily.

Recently, evidence has emerged that standard immunohistochemical markers can have a predictive value similar to the RS. In a study of 1,125 patients from the ATAC trial, a comparison of the Oncotype DX with the IHC4 score (a formula utilizing four standard immunohistochemical markers: ER, PR, Ki67, and HER2) showed that all four IHC markers provided independent prognostic information in the presence of classical variables (Cuzick et al. 2011). The information from the IHC4 score was similar to that in the RS, and little additional prognostic value was seen in the combined use of both scores. These preliminary results suggest that four standard IHC assays performed in a high quality laboratory can provide prognostic information similar to the RS for endocrine-treated ER-positive breast cancer patients. However, additional studies are required to determine the reproducibility and general applicability of this test.

A formal integration of the RS and the classic pathologic and clinical factors, such as tumor size, tumor grade, and patient age, has been performed and will soon be available online (Tang et al. 2010, 2011). In this meta-analysis, which included 647 patients from NSABP B-14 and 1,088 patients from the ATAC trial, the risk of distant recurrence was assessed by using the RS, pathologic factors, and clinical information. These disparate sources of information were then combined to derive the RS-pathology-clinical (RSPC) assessment of distant recurrence risk. The RSPC model provided significantly improved prognostic results for distant recurrence risk compared with the RS alone ($p < 0.001$), or compared with a model using tumor grade, size, and patient age ($p < 001$). Compared with the RS alone, there was an improved separation of risk, with a 33 % relative reduction in the number of patients with intermediate RS (17.8 % for RSPC vs. 26.7 % for RS, $p < 0.001$) and an 18 % relative increase in the number of patients with a low RS (63.8 % for RSPC vs. 54.2 % for RS, $p < 0.001$). This RSPC model will likely have its greatest utility in these low- and intermediate-risk patients.

An association has been demonstrated between the RS and the risk of locoregional recurrence (LRR) (Mamounas et al. 2010). The study analyzed 895 tamoxifen-treated patients from the NSABP B-14 and B-20 trials, 355 placebo-treated patients from B-14, and 424 chemotherapy and tamoxifen-treated patients from B-20. The primary endpoint was the time to first LRR. In the tamoxifen-treated patients, the risk of LRR was significantly correlated with the RS-risk groups ($p < 0.001$). The 10-year estimate of LRR was 4.3 % for the low-risk, 7.2 % for the intermediate-risk, and 15.8 % for the high-risk RS groups. There was also a significant association between LRR and the RS in the placebo-treated group ($p = 0.022$) and the chemotherapy and tamoxifen-treated group ($p = 0.028$). These results are not surprising given the strong associations between LRR and distant recurrence, and they may be helpful in making clinical decisions regarding locoregional therapy.

The use of the 21-gene RS assay can have an impact on both physician and patient decisions about adjuvant therapy. A multicenter study was conducted to prospectively determine whether the RS affects physician and patient adjuvant treatment selection and satisfaction (Lo et al. 2010). Physician adjuvant treatment recommendations were assessed before and after obtaining the RS in 89 assessable patients. Patients were also asked about their treatment choices before and after the RS was obtained, and measures of decisional conflict, anxiety and quality of life were assessed. In 28 patients (31.5 %), the recommendation of the medical oncologist was changed when the RS score was provided. The largest change was from a pretest recommendation of chemotherapy plus hormonal therapy to a post-test recommendation of hormonal therapy only. This occurred in 20 patients (22.5 %). Nine patients (10.1 %) changed their treatment decision from chemotherapy and hormonal therapy to hormonal therapy only. Medical oncologists reported an increased confidence in their treatments in 68 cases (76 %). Patient anxiety and decisional conflict were significantly lower after RS results were provided.

Similar results have been shown across six other independent decision impact studies (Asad et al. 2008; Henry et al. 2009; Klang et al. 2010; Liang et al. 2007; Oratz et al. 2007; Thanasoulis et al. 2008). A meta-analysis of these studies included a total of 912 patient from both academic and community centers in the United States and showed that there was a consistently large impact of the RS on treatment decisions in both directions (Hornberger and Chien 2010, 2011). Overall, the RS led to a 37 % change in treatment decisions. In 52 % of patients, there was a switch from the initial recommendation of chemotherapy and hormonal therapy to hormonal therapy alone and in 12 % of patients, there was a switch from the initial recommendation of hormonal therapy alone to chemotherapy and hormonal therapy. Results from this meta-analysis underscore a consistent and large impact of the RS on treatment decisions by physicians. Recommendations changed in more than a third of treatment decisions after integrating the RS information with traditional measures.

In addition to RS, Genomic Health also includes the results of ER, PR, and HER2 testing by RT-PCR assessment in their reports. A study of 776 breast cancer patients from the Eastern Cooperative Oncology Group (ECOG) E2197 compared ER and PR measured by local laboratory immunohistochemistry (IHC), central IHC, and central reverse-transcriptase polymerase chain reaction (RT-PCR) using the 21-gene assay. There was a high degree of concordance between the three assays (84–93 %) (Badve et al. 2008).

Although ER expression was marginally associated with relapse in ER-positive patients treated with chemotherapy and hormonal therapy, the RS was a highly significant predictor of recurrence in these patients. Despite this excellent concordance, evidence showing the prognostic and predictive value of the qRT-PCR cutoffs to define positivity is still awaited. A study comparing central laboratory HER2 testing by fluorescence in situ hybridization (FISH) to RT-PCR in lymph node-negative, chemotherapy-untreated patients from a large Kaiser Permanente case–control study showed that HER2 concordance by central FISH and central RT-PCR was 97 % (95 % CI, 96–99 %) (Baehner et al. 2010). In contrast, in an independent quality assurance study of 843 patient cases comparing local FISH testing for HER2 to available HER2 RT-PCR results from Genomic Health, there was an high false-negative rate for HER2 status with the RT-PCR assay (Dabbs et al. 2011). Therefore, RT-PCR-based assessments of ER, PR and HER2 should be interpreted together with the results of the FDA-approved methods for assessment of these biomarkers.

The role of gene expression profiling in the treatment of ductal carcinoma in situ (DCIS) has recently been evaluated. A new, prespecified DCIS Score was analyzed to predict recurrence in patients from the ECOG 5194 trial (Solin et al. 2011). In that trial, 670 eligible patients with low- or intermediate-grade DCIS ≤ 2.5 cm or high-grade DCIS ≤ 1 cm were treated with surgical excision only, without radiation, and 228 received tamoxifen (Hughes et al. 2009). RT-PCR analysis was performed in 327 patients (49 % of the original population). The primary objective was to determine whether there was a significant association between the risk of an ipsilateral breast event (IBE) and the continuous DCIS Score. With a median follow-up of 8.8 years, the study was able to prospectively validate that the DCIS score quantifies recurrence risk and complements traditional clinical and pathologic factors.

Prospective clinical trials to evaluate the 21-gene RT-PCR assay are ongoing. The TAILORx trial has completed accrual, but the results have not yet been reported. This is the largest randomized adjuvant trial ever conducted, enrolling over 10,000 patients. All of the patients had the 21-gene RT-PCR assay performed, and those with a RS between 11 and 25 were randomized to either hormonal therapy alone or hormonal therapy with chemotherapy. Patients with a RS ≤ 10 were treated with hormonal therapy only and those with a RS > 25 were given chemotherapy and hormonal therapy. The RS ranges for this trial have been altered from the original definitions of low, intermediate, and high risk to minimize potential for undertreatment in the high- and intermediate-risk groups. Another trial, the RxPONDER trial, also known as SWOG S1007, was opened in January 2011 and is currently accruing patients. The study will randomize 4,000 patients with early-stage, hormone receptor-positive, HER2-negative breast cancer with 1–3 positive lymph nodes who have an RS of ≤ 25 to receive either chemotherapy plus endocrine therapy or endocrine therapy alone. Patients will be stratified into groups by RS 0–13 versus 14–25, by menopausal status, and by axillary lymph node dissection versus sentinel lymph node biopsy. Results from both of these trials will help to further validate the RS and to more clearly define the role of the 21-gene RT-PCR assay in the node-positive population.

4   70 Gene Signature (MammaPrint)

The 70-gene signature (MammaPrint) is a purely prognostic assay for women less than 61 years of age with node-negative, ER-positive, or ER-negative breast cancer. Outside of the United States, it is also being used for patients with 1–3 positive nodes. This test uses DNA microarray technology to determine gene expression, using fresh frozen tumor samples. It can also be performed on formalin-fixed, paraffin-embedded tissue, although the data validating this technique are limited.

The assay focuses on genes involved in proliferation and also measures genes regulating invasion, metastases, stromal integrity, and angiogenesis. It does not directly assess ER, PR, or HER2. The test gives dichotomous results, predicting either a high or low risk of disease recurrence. A correlation coefficient is calculated between a patient's expression levels of the 70 genes and an average good-prognosis expression profile. If the correlation coefficient exceeds 0.4, the patient is classified as having a good-prognosis signature, whereas a coefficient less than 0.4 is classified as a poor-prognosis signature.

In 2007, the 70-gene signature test received approval by the FDA as a prognostic test for breast cancer patients less than 61 years, with tumors less than 5 cm, node-negative and stage I or II breast cancer (Harris et al. 2007). It is approved for both ER-positive and ER-negative disease, but its use in ER-negative disease is limited by the fact that less than 10 % of those tumors will have a good-prognosis signature. The American Society of Clinical Oncology has determined that definitive recommendations for the use of this assay will require data from more clearly directed retrospective studies or from the ongoing MINDACT Trial which will be discussed later.

The 70-gene signature was developed at the Netherlands Cancer Institute, where investigators performed an analysis of gene expression arrays on frozen tissue from 98 sporadic primary breast tumor samples (van't Veer et al. 2002). All of the women were less than 55 years old with tumors less than 5 cm and negative lymph nodes. All of the patients were treated with locoregional therapies only. Seventy-eight (80 %) were sporadic cases, 18 had BRCA 1 mutations, and two had BRCA 2 mutations. Of the original 78 sporadic tumors, 34 (44 %) had distant metastases within 5 years, whereas 44 patients (66 %) did not. A set of 231 genes was initially identified and found to be statistically significantly associated with disease outcome, defined as the presence of distant metastases within 5 years. This group of genes was then refined to a core group of 70 genes. This 70-gene set had an 83 % accuracy at differentiating patients who developed distant disease relapse from those who did not. The classifier correctly predicted the disease outcome for 65 of the 78 patients (83 %) with 5 poor-prognosis signature patients. Eight good-prognosis signature patients were assigned incorrectly.

The 70-gene signature assay was then validated in several studies. The first trial was a retrospective analysis that included 295 young patients (age <53 at diagnosis) with T1 or T2 tumors (van de Vijver et al. 2002). Of note, 61 of these node-negative patients were also part of the original study done to establish the 70-gene profile, which has been one of the criticisms of this validation study. Of the 295 patients, 151 patients were node-negative and 144 were node-positive; 69 patients were ER-negative and 226 were ER-positive. Adjuvant treatment was given to 10 of the 151 node-negative patients and 120 of the 144 node-positive patients. The treatment consisted of chemotherapy in 90 patients, hormone therapy in 20 patients, and a combination of both in 20 patients. The patients were followed for nearly 7 years. Good-prognosis signatures were seen in 115 patients and poor-prognosis signatures in 180. Patients with node-negative and node-positive diseases were evenly distributed between the two signature groups, indicating that the prognosis profile was independent of the nodal status. There was a strong correlation between the good-prognosis 70-gene signatures and the absence of death or early distant recurrence. Overall 10-year survival rates were 94.5 ± 2.6 % and 54.6 ± 4.4 %, respectively, for the good- and poor-prognosis signature groups. At 10 years, the probability of remaining free of distant metastases was 85.2 ± 4.3 % in the group with a good-prognosis signature and 50.6 ± 4.5 % in the group with a poor-prognosis signature. The odds ratio (OR) for the development of distant metastases at 5 years in the node-negative patients (excluding the patients that overlapped with the prior study) was 15.3, similar to the result of 15 seen in the previous study. For the node-positive patients, the prognostic signature was also highly significant, with an OR of 13.7, $p < 0.001$. In the multivariate analysis, the poor-prognosis signature was the strongest prognostic factor for the development of distant metastases. The prognosis profile was significantly associated with histological grade ($p < 0.001$), ER status ($p < 0.001$), and age ($p < 0.001$) but not with tumor size, extent of vascular invasion, number of lymph nodes involved or the treatment given. This study also evaluated the node-negative patients after they were divided into risk categories based on clinical-pathological criteria using the St. Gallen criteria (Goldhirsch et al. 2001) and the NIH criteria (Eifel et al. 2001). The gene signature profile assigned more patients to the low-risk or good-prognosis signature groups than traditional methods did: 40 % for the 70-gene assay, 15 % for the St. Gallen criteria, and 17 % for the NIH criteria. The low-risk patients, identified by a good-prognosis signature, had a higher likelihood of metastasis-free survival than those identified as low risk by the St. Gallen or NIH criteria. In addition, the patients identified as high risk by a poor-prognosis signature tended to have a higher rate of distant metastases than did patients identified as high risk by the St. Gallen or NIH criteria. This led to the conclusion that clinical–pathological criteria could misclassify a significant number of patients and could thus result in many patients being either over-treated or under-treated. In this study, the 70-gene signature was the strongest prognostic factor for distant metastasis-free survival, independent of adjuvant treatment, tumor size, lymph node status, histological grade, or age.

A second study was an independent validation of the 70-gene signature in 307 women, less than 60 years of age, with node-negative, T1 or T2 primary tumors who had not been treated with adjuvant systemic therapy (Buyse et al. 2006). The median follow-up was 13.6 years. Frozen samples were available for the 70-gene signature analysis, and the tumors were scored as low or high risk. The tumors were also assigned to clinical risk categories based on adjuvant! online criteria (patient age, comorbidities, tumor size, tumor grade, ER status, and nodal involvement) (Adjuvant!! Inc. 2012). The authors determined that the low-clinical risk group would be defined as patients with a 10-year overall survival probability of at least 88 %, if 10 % or more of the tumor cells expressed detectable ER, or of at least 92 %, if ER expression was seen in less than 10 % of the tumor cells. When adjusted for clinical risk groups based on the 10-year survival probability as calculated by adjuvant!, the 70-gene signature performed independently of clinical variables in predicting time to distant metastases (HR 2.13, 95 % CI 1.19–3.82) and overall survival (HR 2.63, 95 % CI 1.45–4.79), but not disease-free survival. High-risk patients had a 10-year overall survival of 70 % compared to 90 % for those with low-risk signatures. This study showed that the 70-gene signature provides prognostic information independent of the traditional clinical and pathological risk factors in patients with early-stage breast cancer untreated with systemic therapy.

A third validation study evaluated 123 patients less than 55 years of age with T1-2 N0 breast cancer diagnosed between 1996 and 1999, with a median follow-up of 5.8 years (Bueno-de-Mesquita et al. 2009). Adjuvant treatment was given to 45 patients (37 %): 18 (15 %) received

chemotherapy, 14 (11 %) received endocrine therapy, and 13 (11 %) received both. Good-prognosis signatures were seen in 52 % and poor-prognosis signatures in 48 % of patients. The poor-prognosis signatures were associated with larger tumors, higher histological grade, and ER-negative and PR-negative status. The 5-year overall survival was 97 ± 2 % for the good-prognosis signatures and 82 ± 5 % for the poor-prognosis signatures, HR 3.4, 95 % CI 1.2–9.6, $p = 0.021$. The 5-year distant metastasis (as first event)-free percentage was 98 ± 2 % for the good-prognosis and 78 ± 6 % for the poor-prognosis signatures, HR 5.7, 95 % CI 1.6–2.0, $p = 0.007$. In a multivariate analysis, the prognosis signature was an independent prognostic factor and outperformed the clinical and pathological criteria.

There are clinical data to suggest that the 70-gene signature can predict the response to chemotherapy, although this has not been sufficiently validated for clinical use. In one study, 167 patients with stage I–III breast cancer were analyzed prior to neoadjuvant chemotherapy, and the rate of pathological complete response (pCR) was used to measure chemosensitivity (Straver et al. 2010). Good-prognosis signatures were seen in 23 patients (14 %) and poor-prognosis signatures in 144 patients (86 %). All 38 of the triple-negative (ER-, PR-, and HER2-negative) patients had poor-prognosis signatures. Pathologic complete responses were seen in 29 of the 144 patients with poor-prognosis signatures and in none of the 23 patients with good-prognosis signatures, $p = 0.015$. The authors concluded that the patients with poor-prognosis signatures were more sensitive to chemotherapy. Two other studies have also shown that patients with poor-prognosis signatures are more likely to achieve an excellent pathological response with neoadjuvant chemotherapy than those tumors expressing a good-prognosis profile (Esserman et al. 2009; Pusztai et al. 2008). Another study showed a significant survival benefit for the addition of adjuvant chemotherapy in patients with the poor-prognosis signature but not for those with a good-prognosis signature (Knauer et al. 2010). In 541 patients, the 70-gene signature classified 252 patients (47 %) as low risk and 289 (53 %) as high risk. Within the low-risk group, there was no significant difference in the 5-year breast cancer-specific survival (BCSS) between patients who received endocrine therapy alone and those who received chemotherapy and endocrine therapy, 97 % versus 99 %, $p = 0.62$. In the high-risk group, the 5-year BCSS was 81 % for those who received endocrine therapy and 94 % for the endocrine therapy and chemotherapy, $p < 0.01$. Similarly, distant disease-free survival (DDFS) at 5 years was not significantly different for endocrine therapy alone or endocrine therapy with chemotherapy for the low-risk group (93 % vs. 99 %, $p = 0.20$), whereas it was significantly better for the high-risk patients with the addition of chemotherapy (76 % vs. 88 %, $p < 0.01$).

The 70-gene signature has been evaluated in other groups of breast cancer patients, including postmenopausal women, and patients with positive lymph nodes. In one study, 148 patients aged 55–70 with T1-2 N0 tumors were analyzed, and 91 (61 %) were found to have good risk, while 57 (39 %) had poor-risk signatures (Mook et al. 2010). In these patients, the BCSS at 5 years was 99 and 80 % for the good and poor-risk groups, respectively ($p = 0.036$). The distant metastasis-free survival rates were 93 and 72 %, respectively. The 70-gene prognosis signature was a significant and independent predictor of BCSS during the first 5 years of follow-up with an adjusted hazard ratio (HR) of 14.4 (95 % confidence interval 1.7–122.2; $P = 0.01$) at 5 years. These patients were also analyzed by adjuvant! criteria, which identified 74 patients (50 %) as clinical low risk and 74 patients (50 %) as clinical high risk. There was disagreement with the genomic prognosis in 41 (28 %) patients. Twelve (8 %) patients were identified as clinical low risk but had poor-prognosis genomic signatures, and 29 (28 %) of patients were clinical high risk but had good-prognosis signatures. This study validated the prognostic utility of the 70-gene signature in postmenopausal women and showed that its greatest strength was in the first 5 years after diagnosis. The authors concluded that the beneficial effects of chemotherapy in postmenopausal women occur mostly in the first 5 years after diagnosis and the accurate identification of patients who will have early events, using this signature, may be helpful in selecting patients for adjuvant chemotherapy. A second study retrospectively evaluated 100 postmenopausal patients (median age 62.5) with node-negative disease with the 70-gene signature and adjuvant! online criteria (Wittner et al. 2008) In this study, 27 patients were identified as low risk by the 70-gene signature. None of these patients had distant metastasis as a first event, leading to a negative predictive value of 100 %. Seventy-three patients were identified as high risk by the 70-gene signature. Of these, 9 had distant metastasis as the first event and the other 64 did not. This led to a positive predictive value of 12 %, which was lower than had previously been observed. In comparison with adjuvant! online, the 70-gene signature identified an additional 21 patients as low risk, and none of these patients developed a distant metastasis as the first event.

The 70-gene signature has been shown to have prognostic value in node-positive disease as well. In one of the original validation studies, 144 of the 295 patients had node-positive disease (van de Vijver et al. 2002). Fifty-five of the patients had good-prognosis and 89 had poor-prognosis signatures, and the 70-gene prognostic signature was highly predictive of the risk of distant metastases in these node-positive patients. Although nodal involvement is considered to be predictive of poorer survival, this analysis demonstrated that there is a group of patients who may have a favorable prognosis, despite having positive axillary nodes.

In another study of node-positive patients, 241 patients with T1 to operable T3 tumors with 1–3 positive axillary lymph nodes, including those with micrometastases, were analyzed using the 70-gene signature (Mook et al. 2009). The patients received local treatment followed by adjuvant systemic therapy, according to national guidelines and patient preferences. The 70-gene signature was performed, and clinical risk assessment was also determined by adjuvant! The 70-gene signature classified 99 (41 %) as good prognosis and 142 (59 %) as poor prognosis. The poor-prognosis signature patients were more likely to have received adjuvant chemotherapy, less likely to have received endocrine therapy, and tended to have larger, more poorly differentiated, ER- and PR-negative, and HER2-positive tumors. Breast cancer-specific survival (BCSS) at 5 years was 99 % for the good-prognosis signature vs. 80 % for the poor-prognosis signature group ($P = 0.036$). The 10-year distant metastasis-free survival (DMFS) and BCSS were 91 and 96 % for the good-prognosis signature group and 76 and 76 % for the poor-prognosis signature group. Using adjuvant! online, 32 patients (13 %) were classified as clinical low risk and 209 (87 %) were classified as clinical high risk. The clinical risk category was discordant with the 70-gene prognosis signature in 77 patients (32 %): 5 patients were identified as clinical low-risk with a poor-prognosis signature, whereas 72 were classified as clinical high-risk with a good-prognosis signature. For the 209 patients identified as clinical high risk, the 10-year BCSS was 94 % for those in the good-prognosis signature group and 76 % for those in the poor-prognosis signature group. In the 27 patients classified as low risk by both the adjuvant! online criteria and the 70-gene signature, none developed distant metastatic disease or died. Again, the 70-gene prognosis signature outperformed traditional prognostic factors in predicting disease outcome in patients in this population and accurately identified some patients with 1–3 positive nodes who had a favorable outcome.

The original 70-gene signature was generated on microarrays that were not designed for processing of many samples on a routine basis. To improve its clinical utility, a customized microarray (marketed as MammaPrint) with a reduced set of probes was developed. One study re-analyzed the 145 patients from the original validation study (van de Vijver et al. 2002) and the 78 patients from the training set (van't Veer et al. 2002), compared the results from the original analysis to the custom microarray, and found an extremely high correlation of prognostic prediction between the two assays ($p < 0.0001$) (Glas et al. 2006).

Currently, a large prospective randomized trial, the MINDACT, is being conducted in Europe. This study compares the 70-gene signature to the traditional clinical and pathological criteria used to select patients for adjuvant chemotherapy. The trial opened in February 2007, and the plan is to enroll 6,000 early-stage breast cancer patients (T1, T2, and operable T3M0). Originally, the study included only node-negative patients, but more recently, it was expanded to include patients with 1–3 positive lymph nodes. The patients are assessed by the standard clinicopathologic prognostic factors included in adjuvant! and by the 70-gene signature assay. If both traditional and molecular assays predict a high-risk status, then the patient will receive adjuvant cytotoxic chemotherapy (and hormonal therapy if the tumor is ER-positive). If both assays indicate a low risk, no chemotherapy is given and ER-positive patients are given adjuvant hormonal therapy only. When there is discordance between the traditional clinicopathologic prognostic factors and the 70-gene signature, patients are randomized to receive treatment based on either the genomic or the clinical predictive results. The results of this trial will provide more data about the use of the 70-gene signature in early-stage breast cancer.

5 The HOXB13:IL17BR Ratio

The anti-apoptotic homeobox B13 (HOXB13) gene and interleukin 17 B receptor (IL17BR) gene are used to calculate the HOXB13:IL17BR (H/I) expression ratio. This ratio was developed by a microarray-based screening of 22,000 genes in 60 patients with ER-positive, node-positive, or node-negative breast cancer, treated with tamoxifen (Ma et al. 2004). Three genes that were identified were significantly associated with clinical outcome: HOXB13, IL17BR, and CHDH (choline dehydrogenase). High expression of HOXB13 was associated with recurrence, while high expression of IL17BR and CHDH was associated with non-recurrence. A higher ratio of the HOXB13 and IL17BR strongly predicted recurrence, and pairing with CHDH did not provide additional predictive power. A larger validation study was done in 852 patients with stage I or II breast cancer with a median follow-up of 6.8 years (Ma et al. 2006). In this study, 286 (34 %) patients were tamoxifen-treated and 566 (66 %) patients were untreated. Of note, patients were not randomized to a treatment arm. The expression of HOXB13, IL17BR, and CHDH, as well as ER and PR were quantified by RT-PCR. Gene expression and clinical variables were analyzed for association with relapse-free survival. Expression of HOXB13 was associated with a shorter RFS ($p = 0.008$), whereas the expression of IL17BR and CHDH was associated with longer RFS ($p < 0.0001$ and $p = 0.0002$, respectively). In the ER-positive patients, the HOXB13:IL17BR index predicted clinical outcome, independently of treatment, but more strongly in the node-negative patients. This study also suggested a role for the H/I ratio as a prognostic test in untreated patients. The HOXB13/IL17BR ratio was tested but not verified in a retrospective study of 58 ER-positive patients treated with tamoxifen for 5 years, most of whom were node-positive (77 %) (Reid et al. 2005). In this study, the H/I ratio failed to show a relationship between the expression of these genes and distant relapse or survival.

The association between the H/I ratio and clinical outcome was evaluated in tumor specimens from the NCCTG 89-30-52 trial (Goetz et al. 2006). In this trial, postmenopausal women with ER-positive breast cancer were randomized to 5 years of tamoxifen with or without 1 year of fluoxymesterone. For the 227 patients in the tamoxifen-only arm, RT-PCR profiles for HOXB13 and IL17BR were obtained from 206 paraffin-embedded tumor blocks. In the node-positive cohort ($n = 86$), the H/I ratio was not associated with relapse or survival. In contrast, in the node-negative cohort ($n = 130$), a high H/I ratio was associated with a significantly decreased relapse-free survival [HR, 1.98; $P = 0.031$], disease-free survival (HR, 2.03; $P = 0.015$), and overall survival (HR, 2.4; $P = 0.014$), independent of standard prognostic markers. One explanation could be that these genes may have a role in early invasion and metastatic potential, and therefore, they could be more relevant in the node-negative population. Similar findings regarding the nodal status were demonstrated in a large cohort ($N = 852$) of both untreated and tamoxifen-treated patients (Erlander et al. 2005). In this study, the H/I ratio was associated with relapse and death in node-negative but not node-positive, ER-positive patients.

In another study, the ability of the H/I ratio to predict disease-free survival was tested in 1,252 breast tumor specimens (Jansen et al. 2007). In 468 patients with node-negative, ER-positive breast cancer who did not receive adjuvant chemotherapy, the H/I ratio was significantly associated with poorer disease-free survival (HR, 1.6; $P = 0.02$) and poorer overall survival (HR not reported; $P < 0.001$). In a multivariate analysis of 151 untreated patients with ER-positive, node-positive breast cancer, an association was shown between the H/I ratio and overall survival ($p < 0.001$) but not disease-free survival ($p = 0.065$). In 193 patients treated with tamoxifen at first relapse, the ratio was significantly associated with progression-free survival. The authors concluded that higher H/I ratio expression levels are associated with both tumor aggressiveness and failure to respond to tamoxifen. One study investigated whether the H/I ratio predicted a difference in benefit between 264 patients with postmenopausal breast cancer who received tamoxifen for 2 and 5 years and 93 pre-menopausal patients who did not receive systemic therapy (Jerevall et al. 2008). In this study, 72 % of the patients had node-positive disease and 74 % had ER-positive disease. The HOXB13:IL17BR gene expression ratio and the expression of HOXB13 alone predicted the benefit of endocrine therapy, with a high ratio or a high expression rendering patients less likely to respond. Neither the patient profile nor the methods of calculation of the ratio were identical to those used in previous studies. The results of this study differed from previous reports because, in this case, the H/I ratio was associated with outcomes in patients with lymph node-positive disease.

6 Theros Breast Cancer Index

Theros Breast Cancer Index (TBCI) is a prognostic profile that provides a quantitative assessment of the likelihood of distant recurrence in patients with ER-positive, node-negative breast cancer. It is a molecular assay that combines two indices—HOXB13:IL17BR and a five-gene molecular grade index (MGI). The MGI is a gene expression index for tumor grade that includes 5 cell cycle-related genes. It was generated using two microarray data sets testing a total of 410 patients (Ma et al. 2008). A 323-patient cohort was used to develop an RT-PCR assay for MGI and to validate its prognostic utility. When combined with the HOXB13:IL17BR index, it was noted that the two assays modified the prognostic performance of each other. A high MGI was associated with a significantly worse outcome only in combination with a high HOXB13:IL17BR, and likewise, a high HOXB13:IL17BR was significantly associated with a poor outcome only in combination with a high MGI.

The TBCI was further assessed in a retrospective study of 262 patients with ER-positive, node-negative breast cancer with at least a 10-year follow-up (Jankowitz et al. 2010). The TBCI was compared to adjuvant! online to see whether it added additional predictive power for recurrence and overall survival. The TBCI predicted breast cancer recurrence and overall survival more accurately than adjuvant! online combined with and traditional clinical and pathologic features. Both TBCI and adjuvant! online retained independent prognostic significance for recurrence and death in a multivariate analysis, indicating that the two tests can provide complementary information.

7 Rotterdam 76-Gene Signature

A 76-gene signature was developed using 286 tumor samples of node-negative breast cancers from a single institution (Wang et al. 2005). In a training set of 115 tumors, gene expression analysis led to the identification of a 76-gene signature consisting of 60 genes for ER-positive tumors and 16 genes for ER-negative tumors. The 76-gene signature showed 93 % sensitivity and 48 % specificity in a subsequent independent testing set of 171 lymph node-negative patients. The gene profile identified patients who developed distant metastases within 5 years (HR 5.67 [95 % CI 2.59–12.4]), even when corrected for the traditional prognostic factors in a multivariate analysis (5.55 [2.46–12.5]). After 5 years, the absolute differences in distant metastasis-free and overall survival between the patients with the good or poor 76-gene signatures were 40 and 27 %, respectively. Among the patients with good-prognosis signatures, 7 % developed distant metastases and 3 % died within 5 years. The 76-gene profile also provided significant prognostic information regarding the development of metastasis in premenopausal patients (84 patients), postmenopausal patients (87 patients), and patients with tumors measuring 10–20 mm. In this series, the assay also outperformed the St. Gallen's (Goldhirsch et al. 2001, 2005) and NIH guidelines (NIH Consensus Statement Online 2000; Eifel et al. 2001) for the identification of patients with a good prognosis.

The 76-gene signature profile was further validated in an independent multicenter study of 180 patients with node-negative breast cancer who did not receive adjuvant systemic therapy (Foekens et al. 2006). In this study, frozen samples were analyzed by quantitative RT-PCR rather than microarray analysis. The 76-gene signature was highly accurate in identifying patients who would develop distant metastasis within 5 years (HR, 7.41; 95 % CI, 2.63–20.9), even when corrected for traditional prognostic factors in a multivariate analysis (HR, 11.36; 95 % CI, 2.67–48.4). The actuarial 5- and 10-year distant metastasis-free survival rates were 96 % (95 % CI, 89–99 %) and 94 % (95 % CI, 83–98 %), respectively, for the good-profile group and 74 % (95 % CI, 64 % to 81 %) and 65 % (53–74 %), respectively for the poor-profile group. The 76-gene signature was confirmed as a strong prognostic factor in subgroups of ER-positive patients, premenopausal and postmenopausal patients, and patients with tumors that were 20 mm or smaller. The subgroup of patients with ER-negative tumors was too small to perform a separate analysis.

Like the 70-gene signature, this assay requires fresh or frozen tissue, and the prognostic information relies primarily on the degree of expression of proliferation-related genes. It may not be useful in assessing the outcome in patients with ER-negative, HER2-negative cancers (Wirapati et al. 2008; Desmedt et al. 2007).

8 Mammostrat

Mammostrat® is an immunohistochemical (IHC) assay that measures five biomarkers: SLC7A5, HTF9C, P53, NDRG1, and CEACAM5. This test could potentially be implemented in the routine pathologic assessment of breast cancers because it is performed using IHC. The biomarkers are independent of one another and do not directly measure either proliferation or hormone receptor status. They were selected from gene expression data which guided the production of hundreds of novel antibody reagents (Ring et al. 2006). Five reagents (p53, NDRG1, CEACAM5, SLC7A5, and HTF9C) were shown to identify ER-positive patients with poor outcomes. The assay was then tested in a blinded, retrospective study using tissue arrays of paraffin blocks from the ER-positive, node-negative samples from the NSABP B14 and B20 trials (Ross et al. 2008). Tissue arrays were stained by IHC, targeting the 5 biomarkers, and risk stratification was done using predefined scoring rules, an algorithm for combining scores, and cutoff points for low-risk, moderate-risk, and high-risk patient groups. In a multivariate model, the IHC assay contributed information independent of age, tumor size, or menopausal status ($P = 0.007$). The Kaplan–Meier estimates for recurrence-free survival after 10 years were 73, 86, and 85 % for the high-risk, moderate-risk, and low-risk groups ($P = 0.001$), and the breast cancer-specific death rates were 23, 10, and 9 % ($P < 0.0001$), respectively. Both high-risk and low-risk groups showed significant improvement with cytotoxic chemotherapy. However, the magnitude of benefit in the high-risk patients was four times greater than in the low-risk patients. The largest validation of this assay was done in a single institution series from 1981 to 1998. 1,812 women with early-stage breast cancer were studied, and 1,390 cases were assayed (Bartlett et al. 2010). Each case was assigned a Mammostrat® risk score, and distant recurrence-free survival (DRFS), RFS, and overall survival (OS) were analyzed by marker positivity and risk score. An increased Mammostrat® score was significantly associated with reduced DRFS, RFS, and OS in patients with ER-positive breast cancer ($P < 0.00001$). In node-negative, tamoxifen-treated patients, 10-year recurrence rates were 7.6 ± 1.5 % in the low-risk group vs. 20.0 ± 4.4 % in the high-risk group.

9 PAM-50

PAM-50 is a 50-gene assay using quantitative RT-PCR, developed to identify intrinsic breast cancer subtypes (luminal A/B, HER2-enriched, basal-like). It also includes genes related to proliferation and tumor size. It can be performed on archival breast tissue. A risk of relapse (ROR) score is generated for all patients, including those with ER-negative disease. In a test set of 761 patients who did not receive any systemic therapy, the intrinsic subtypes showed prognostic significance ($P = 2.26E-12$) and the results remained significant in multivariable analyses that incorporated standard parameters, including ER status, histological grade, tumor size, and node status (Parker et al. 2009). A combined model of subtype and tumor size was a significant improvement on either the clinical/pathological model or

subtype model alone. In a set of 133 patients treated with neoadjuvant anthracycline and taxanes, the intrinsic subtype model predicted neoadjuvant chemotherapy efficacy with a negative predictive value for pathologic complete response of 97 %.

In a series of 786 patients with ER-positive breast cancer, treated with tamoxifen, the PAM50 qRT-PCR signatures performed on formalin-fixed, paraffin-embedded tissue gave more prognostic information than clinical assays for hormone receptors or Ki-67 (Nielsen et al. 2010). In node-negative patients, PAM50 qRT-PCR-based risk assignment weighted for tumor size and proliferation identified a group with >95 % 10-year survival without chemotherapy. In node-positive patients, PAM50-based prognostic models were also superior.

The PAM50 risk of recurrence (ROR) score was evaluated in the TransATAC population (ER-positive, node-negative, and node-positive women treated with anastrozole or tamoxifen), and compared with the OncotypeDx and a composite IHC score (IHC4), including ER, PR, HER2, and Ki-67 (Dowsett et al. 2011). In this study, PAM-50 provided greater prognostic information than the OncotypeDx RS, and as much information as the IHC4. PAM50 was prognostic for 10-year distant recurrence in the overall population, and in node-positive, node-negative, and HER2-negative patients. Similar results were seen with a 46-gene variation (PAM-46).

10 EndoPredict—11 Genes

The EndoPredict (EP) assay evaluates eight cancer-related and three reference genes using quantitative RT-PCR on formalin-fixed, paraffin-embedded tissue (Filipits et al. 2011). A risk score is calculated, and the score is either low or high. The EP score was combined with nodal status and tumor size into a comprehensive risk score–EPclin. The test is designed to assess the risk of distant recurrence in patients with ER-positive, HER2-negative breast cancer treated with endocrine therapy alone. The test was validated using samples from two trials: the Austrian Breast and Colorectal Cancer Study Group (ABCSG)-6 ($n = 378$, tamoxifen-only-treated patients) and ABCSG-8 ($n = 1,324$, patients treated with either tamoxifen for 5 years or tamoxifen for 2 years followed by anastrozole for 3 additional years). In both of these cohorts, the continuous EP was an independent predictor of distant recurrence in multivariate analysis (ABCSG-6 $p = 0.010$, ABCSG-8 $p < 0.001$). The test provided prognostic information independent of, and in addition to, clinicopathologic variables, in particular, adjuvant! online and the Ki-67 labeling index.

11 Genomic Grade Index–97 Genes

The genomic grade index (GGI) uses a 97-gene assay to measure the histological tumor grade. The test is based on the premise that the histological grade is a strong prognostic factor in ER-positive tumors, and that the reproducibility of histological grade is suboptimal. The GGI is capable of dividing breast cancers of intermediate grade into two groups, grade I-like, which have a low frequency of distant relapses, and grade III-like, which have a clinical behavior similar to grade III cancers (Sotiriou et al. 2006). Similar results were obtained in an analysis of 347 tumor samples, where it was found that the genomic grade was an independent prognostic indicator of disease recurrence (Ivshina et al. 2006). In another study, 666 ER-positive tumors were classified into high and low genomic grade using the GGI (Loi et al. 2007). These were highly comparable to the previously described luminal A and B classification and significantly correlated with the risk groups generated using the 21-gene RS. The two subtypes were associated with statistically distinct clinical outcome in both tamoxifen-treated and tamoxifen-untreated populations.

The value of the GGI in predicting the response to neoadjuvant chemotherapy in patients with HER-2–normal breast cancer was reported by investigators from the MD Anderson Cancer Center (Liedtke et al. 2009). Gene expression data were generated from fine-needle aspiration biopsies performed on 229 patients prospectively collected before neoadjuvant paclitaxel, fluorouracil, doxorubicin, and cyclophosphamide chemotherapy. Eighty-five percent of grade 1 tumors had low GGI, 89 % of grade 3 tumors had high GGI, and 63 % of grade 2 tumors had low GGI. In both ER-negative and ER-positive patients, a high GGI was associated with a pathologic complete response or minimal residual disease, demonstrating an increased sensitivity to chemotherapy. High GGI was also associated with a significantly worse distant RFS in patients with ER-positive cancer ($p = 0.005$).

Initially, GGI required fresh or frozen samples. However, a modified version of this signature based on qRT-PCR analysis has recently been developed (Toussaint et al. 2009). The prognostic information provided by GGI is applicable only to ER-positive breast cancer (Wirapati et al. 2008; Desmedt et al. 2007).

12 Wound-Response Gene Expression Signature

Core serum response genes are a set of genes closely associated with wound healing and cancer progression. The gene expression profile of fibroblasts activated in the serum is also expressed in tumors by the tumor cells, by tumor-associated fibroblasts, or both. The expression of the wound-response signature was shown to be associated with poor overall survival and an increased risk of metastasis in common epithelial tumors, such as breast, lung, and gastric cancers (Chang et al. 2004). Measurements of genes in this profile show a biphasic pattern of gene expression, with either an activated or quiescent wound-response signature. This profile was validated in the same group of 295 early breast cancer patients that was used to validate the 70-gene signature (Chang et al. 2005). A univariate analysis of the patients showed that the activated signature was associated with a decreased distant metastasis-free and overall survival. The wound-response signature gave more accurate risk stratification independently of known clinical and pathologic risk factors. The 70-gene prognosis signature and intrinsic molecular subtype classification (Perou et al. 2000) were also performed on these tumor samples, and the results from the different gene signatures were overlapping and were all consistent predictors of outcome. Prospective studies are needed to determine whether treatment decisions based on the wound-response signature will benefit patients clinically.

13 Comparison of Different Genetic Profiles

As discussed in this chapter, many studies of gene expression in breast cancer have identified expression profiles and gene sets that are prognostic, predictive, or both. The genes evaluated in these different profiles show only minimal overlap. The reasons for this are not completely understood, but probably include differences in patient cohorts, microarray platforms, and methods of statistical analysis.

There is little data about head-to-head comparisons of the different molecular profiles. However, five profiles were compared in one data set of 295 samples, where information was available about RFS and overall survival (OS). These profiles were the 70-gene signature, the wound-response gene set, the 21-gene RS, the intrinsic subtype model, and the HOXB13/IL17BR two-gene ratio (Fan et al. 2006). These were the same 295 samples that had been used to develop the 70-gene signature (van de Vijver et al. 2002). The RS and two-gene ratio were described as a derived score and estimated from microarray gene expression data rather than qRT-PCR. Therefore, they were not obtained according to the protocols and methods used in the marketed assays. Each of the five gene expression profiles, except for the two-gene ratio, was a significant predictor of RFS and OS, as were ER status, tumor grade, tumor diameter, and stage. This was also true for the 225 tumors that were ER-positive. Each profile, except the two-gene ratio, added important prognostic information beyond the standard clinical predictors.

Table 2 Summary of available prognostic and predictive gene expression signatures

Test	Type of assay	Type of tissue sample	Indication	FDA clearance	ASCO recommended
Oncotype DX	21-gene recurrence score	Formalin-fixed paraffin-embedded	Prognosis and prediction of benefit from chemotherapy in ER+ N0/1–3N+ breast cancer on tamoxifen use	No	Yes
MammaPrint	70-gene signature	Fresh frozen tumor samples	Prognosis in N0, <5 cm tumor diameter, stage I/II, ER± breast cancer	Yes	No
H/I ratio	2-gene expression ratio	Formalin-fixed paraffin-embedded	ER+, N±, stage I/II breast cancer on tamoxifen use	No	No
Theros Breast Cancer Index	Combination of H/I ratio and 5-gene molecular grade index into a breast cancer index	Formalin-fixed paraffin-embedded	Prognosis and prediction of response to tamoxifen in ER+ breast cancer	No	No
EndoPredict	11-gene score	Formalin-fixed paraffin-embedded	ER+, HER2− breast cancer treated with endocrine therapy	No	No
Genomic grade index	97-gene genomic grade index	Frozen or formalin-fixed paraffin-embedded	ER+, histological grade II breast cancer	No	No
Rotterdam 76-gene signature	76-gene signature	Fresh frozen tumor samples	ER±, N0 breast cancer	No	No
Mammostrat	Immunohistochemical assay measuring five biomarkers	Formalin-fixed paraffin-embedded	ER+, N0 breast cancer	No	No
PAM-50	50-gene signature	Formalin-fixed paraffin-embedded	Prognosis in ER+, N ± breast cancer	No	No

Estrogen receptor (ER); Lymph node (N)

Each profile was analyzed relative to the intrinsic subtype classification. All 53 tumors with basal-like subtype were found to have a poor 70-gene signature profile and a high RS, and 50 tumors had an activated wound-response signature. This was also true for the tumors with the HER2-positive, ER-negative subtypes, as well as for the poor-outcome luminal B subtype that is classified as ER positive. Conversely, the normal-like and luminal A tumors showed heterogeneity in terms of how they were classified by the other models. However, 62 of 70 samples with low RS were of the luminal A subtype. These results suggest that if a sample is classified as basal-like, HER2-positive, and ER-negative, or luminal B, then it would most likely be in the poor-prognosis groups of the 70-gene, wound-response, and recurrence score models. Pairwise comparisons of the 70-gene, wound-response, recurrence score, and two-gene models showed that the results of all but the two-gene model were highly concordant. Since the 70-gene signature and the RS model are the best validated, they were directly compared, with low and intermediate RSs considered equivalent to a good 70-gene signature and a high RS to be equivalent to a poor 70-gene signature. In the entire group of patients,

there was 81 % agreement (239/295 patients), and in the ER-positive subset, there was a 77 % agreement (173/225 patients). These results suggest that even though there is very little overlap in the genes that are analyzed (the 70-gene and the RS profiles overlapped by only 1 gene: *SCUBE2*) and different algorithms are used, the outcome predictions provided by these profiles are similar for the majority of patients. The profiles probably reflect common cellular phenotypes and biological characteristics in the different groups of breast cancer patients.

In a comprehensive meta-analysis integrating both clinical, pathological, and gene expression data in over 2,100 patients, a multivariate analysis showed that in the ER+/HER2− subgroup, only the proliferation module and the histological grade were significantly associated with clinical outcome (Desmedt et al. 2008). In the ER−/HER2− subgroup, only the immune response module was associated with prognosis, whereas in the HER2+ tumors, the tumor invasion and immune response modules displayed a significant association with survival. Proliferation was identified as the most important component of the prognostic signatures, and the performance was limited to the ER+/HER2-

subgroup. In another meta-analysis of 2,833 breast cancers, gene coexpression modules of three key biological processes (proliferation, ER signaling and HER2 signaling) were used to analyze the genes of nine prognostic signatures (Wirapati et al. 2008). All nine prognostic signatures had a similar prognostic performance in the entire data set, mostly due to the detection of proliferation activity. In this study, ER status and ERBB2 expression seemed to correspond with a poor outcome, due to elevated expression of proliferation genes. Also, clinical variables, such as tumor size and nodal status, added additional independent prognostic information (Table 2).

14   Limitations

The gene expression prognostic signatures share several characteristics (Reis-Filho and Pusztai 2011). Despite the differences in the genes they measure, the gene signature tests identify the same group of patients as having a poor prognosis. The unifying characteristic is the high expression of proliferation-related genes (Wirapati et al. 2008). When gene signatures were divided into two subsignatures (Wirapati et al. 2008; Reyal et al. 2008) one composed of only the proliferation-related genes and the other composed of the remaining genes, the proliferation-related subsignatures had a prognostic impact as strong or stronger than the original signatures (Wirapati et al. 2008; Reyal et al. 2008). Importantly, the subsignatures composed of non-proliferation-related genes were shown not to have a prognostic impact (Wirapati et al. 2008). This is especially true in ER-positive breast cancers, where the level of expression of proliferation-related genes is one of the strongest prognostic factors. In ER-negative cancers, the expression of proliferation-related genes is usually high and, therefore, gene signatures have failed to stratify ER-negative breast cancers into separate prognostic subgroups (Mook et al. 2009, 2010; Wirapati et al. 2008). Even adenoid cystic carcinoma of the breast, which is ER-negative and has an indolent clinical course, is classified by gene signatures as having a poor prognosis (Weigelt et al. 2008). Chemotherapy targets rapidly proliferating cells, and since the gene signatures predominantly measure proliferation-related genes, most of the gene signature assays also correlate with response to chemotherapy. In addition, meta-analyses have shown that tumor size and lymph node status provide prognostic information that is independent of the results from the prognostic signatures. The accuracy of the predictions of the prognostic signatures seems to be time-dependent, with more accurate predictions seen at 5 years than at 10 years after diagnosis.

The genetic profiles use a variety of techniques to perform the assays in the reported studies. All studies of 21-gene RT-PCR assay have used the commercial test as opposed to the signature, whereas the studies of the 70-gene signature have used either the signature or the assay. Only the large multicenter validation by (Buyse et al. 2006) used the marketed MammaPrint assay. The study that compared the results of the marketed MammaPrint test to the signature on the same samples showed that about 9 % of the patients were placed into different risk groups when the marketed test was used (Glas et al. 2006). Almost all of the studies that looked at the H/I ratio calculated the test in slightly different ways.

The accurate use of these tests in clinical decision making will be vitally important. Only the 21-gene RS has been shown to be prognostic as well as predictive for a benefit from both tamoxifen and chemotherapy. This was based on data from the randomized, clinical trials, NSABP B-14 and B-20 (Paik et al. 2004, 2006). The other genomic tests are purely prognostic and indicate the likely outcome, independent of therapy. These tests have limited data regarding their predictive abilities, but it is assumed that patients who have a low risk of recurrence or death may forgo chemotherapy.

The study populations that were used to validate the various gene signature tests were not uniform. The 21-gene RS used the most clinically and therapeutically homogeneous population. This is reflected in the inclusion criteria for the test: patients with ER-positive, lymph node-negative, stage I or II disease who receive tamoxifen. The 70-gene signature was tested in a more heterogeneous population, with both lymph node-positive and lymph node-negative patients, and patients with ER-positive and ER-negative diseases.

15   Conclusion

In early-stage breast cancer, the standard approach has been to use clinical and pathological variables, such as tumor size, lymph node metastases, tumor grade, ER, PR, and HER2 status to create treatment guidelines (e.g., adjuvant! online, the NCCN guidelines, the NIH Consensus Development Criteria, and the St. Gallen criteria). These guidelines provide risk classifications which help guide decisions regarding adjuvant therapy. These approaches have been successful, and there has been a steady reduction in breast cancer mortality over the past three decades. However, with the development of individualized medicine, genomic signatures can provide a more accurate assessment of the risk of recurrence and the benefit of adjuvant therapy.

Recently, many gene expression profiles have been developed for breast cancer. Several of these tests are now commercially available, and more new tests are being developed. These gene expression profiles appear to provide additional prognostic and predictive information that complements the traditional clinical and pathological parameters. However, most of the genetic profiles have not been validated in prospective randomized trials. Also, there have not been any large, prospective, head-to-head comparisons between the different tests. Each test looks at a different set of genes, and there is little overlap in the tested genes. Despite the lack of overlap, these tests identify the same group of patients as having a poor prognosis, probably because all of the signatures rely heavily on proliferation-related genes (Wirapati et al. 2008). The tests are often only informative in ER-positive breast cancers, which limits their utility. Also, the tests are expensive and may have limited availability.

With so many tests available or in development, some important questions need to be answered: Is the test accurate and reliable? Does the evidence show that it is strongly prognostic? Is there evidence that the test result is predictive of chemotherapy benefit? What is the level of evidence for the accuracy of the assay? Has the assay been incorporated into treatment guidelines?

In spite of all these caveats, the new genetic signatures almost uniformly allow a more accurate prediction of outcomes in breast cancer patients. As the tests are improved, and comparison studies are conducted, the role of the various profiles and the importance of individual genes in the profiles will be better understood. The results from these tests will allow oncologists to spare many women from the toxicities and long-term side effects of unnecessary adjuvant chemotherapy. These multigene assays will contribute to major improvements in the treatment of breast cancer.

References

Adjuvant!! Inc. Adjuvant Online.Decision making tools for health care professionals. Accessed at http://adjuvantonline.com/ on February 10, 2012

Albain KS, Barlow WE, Shak S et al (2010) Prognostic and predictive value of the 21-gene recurrence score assay in postmenopausal women with node-positive, oestrogen-receptor-positive breast cancer on chemotherapy: a retrospective analysis of a randomised trial. Lancet Oncol 11:55–65

American cancer society (2011). Cancer facts and figures 2011. http://www.cancer.org. Accessed December 28, 2011

Asad J, Jacobson A, Estabrook A et al (2008) Does oncotype DX recurrence score affect the management of patients with early stage breast cancer? Am J Surg 196:527–529

Badve SS, Baehner FL, Gray RP et al (2008) Estrogen- and progesterone-receptor status in ECOG 2197: comparison of immunohistochemistry by local and central laboratories and quantitative reverse transcription polymerase chain reaction by central laboratory. J Clin Oncol 26:2473–2481

Baehner FL, Achacoso N, Madalla T et al (2010) Human epidermal growth factor receptor 2 assessment in a case-control study: comparison of fluorescence in situ hybridization and quantitative reverse transcription polymerase chain reaction performed by central laboratories. J Clin Oncol 28:4300–4306

Bartlett JMS, Thomas J, Ross DT et al (2010) Mammostrat as a tool to stratify breast cancer patients at risk of recurrence during endocrine treatment. Breast Cancer Res 2010(12):R47

Bryant J (2005) Toward a more rational selection of tailored adjuvant therapy data from the national surgical adjuvant breast and bowel project. 2005 St. Gallen breast cancer symposium. [Complete slide presentation via genomic health]

Bueno-de-Mesquita JM, Linn SC, Keijzer R et al (2009) Validation of 70-gene prognosis signature in node-negative breast cancer. Breast Cancer Res Treat 117:483–495

Buyse M, Loi S, van't Veer L et al (2006) Validation and clinical utility of a 70-gene prognostic signature for women with node-negative breast cancer. J Natl Cancer Inst 98:1183–1192

Carter CL, Allen C, Henson DE (1989) Relation of tumor size, lymph node status, and survival in 24,740 breast cancer cases. Cancer 63 (1):181–187

Chang HY, Sneddon JB, Alizadeh AA et al (2004) Gene expression signature of fibroblast serum response predicts human cancer progression: similarities between tumors and wounds. PLoSBiol 2: E7–E7

Chang HY, Nuyten DS, Sneddon JB et al (2005) Robustness, scalability, and integration of a wound-response gene expression signature in predicting breast cancer survival. ProcNatlAcadSci USA 102:3738–3743

Chang JC, Makris A, Gutierrez MC et al (2008) Gene expression patterns in formalin-fixed, paraffin-embedded core biopsies predict docetaxel chemosensitivity in breast cancer patients. Breast Cancer Res Treat 108:233–240

Cobleigh MA, Tabesh B, Bitterman P et al (2005) Tumor gene expression and prognosis in breast cancer patients with 10 or more positive lymph nodes. Clin Cancer Res 11:8623–8631

Cuzick J, Dowsett M, Pineda S et al (2011) Prognostic value of a combined estrogen receptor, progesterone receptor, Ki-67 and human epidermal growth factor receptor 2 immunohistochemical score and comparison with the genomic health recurrence score in early breast cancer. J Clin Oncol 29:4273–4278

Dabbs DJ, Klein ME, Mohsin SK et al (2011) High false-negative rate for HER2 quantitative reverse transcription polymerase chain reaction of the OncotypeDx test: an independent quality assurance study. J Clin Oncol 29:4279–4285

Desmedt C, Piette F, Loi S et al (2007) Strong time dependence of the 76-gene prognostic signature for node-negative breast cancer patients in the TRANSBIG multicenter independent validation series. Clin Cancer Res 13:3207–3234

Desmedt C, Haibe-Kains B, Wirapati P et al (2008) Biological processes associated with breast cancer clinical outcome depend on the molecular subtypes. Clin Cancer Res 14:5158–5165

Dowsett M, Cuzick J, Wale C et al (2010) Prediction of risk of distant recurrence using the 21-gene recurrence score in node-negative and node-positive postmenopausal patients with breast cancer treated with anastrozole or tamoxifen: a TransATAC study. J Clin Oncol 28:1829–1834

Dowsett M, Lopez-Knowles E, Sidhu K, et al (2011) Comparison of PAM50 risk of recurrence (ROR) score with OncotypeDx and IHC4 for predicting residual risk of RFS and distant-(D)RFS after endocrine therapy: A TransATAC Study. Antonio breast cancer symposium: 2011: abstract S4-5

Early Breast Cancer Trialists' Collaborative Group (2005) Effects of chemotherapy and hormonal therapy for early breast cancer on recurrence and 15-year survival: an overview of the randomised trials. Lancet 365:1687–1717

Eifel P, Axelson JA, Costa J et al (2001) National institutes of health consensus development conference statement: adjuvant therapy for breast cancer, Nov 1–3, 2000. J Natl Cancer Inst 93(13):979–989

Erlander MG, Ma XJ, Hilsenbeck SG et al (2005) Validation of HOXB13, IL17B and CHDH as predictors of clinical outcome of adjuvant tamoxifen monotherapy in breast cancer. Breast Cancer Res Treat 94:S33–S34

Esserman LJ, Perou C, Cheang A et al (2009) Breast cancer molecular profiles and tumor response of neoadjuvant doxorubicin and paclitaxel: the I-Spy Trial (CALGB 150007/150012, ACRIN 6657). J Clin Oncol 27(suppl):LBA515

Esteban J, Baker J, Cronin M et al (2003) Tumor gene expression and prognosis in breast cancer: multi-gene RT-PCR assay of paraffin-embedded tissue. Proc Am Soc Clin Oncol 22(850):2003 Abstract 3416

Esteva FJ, Sahin AA, Cristofanilli M et al (2005) Prognostic role of a multigene reverse transcriptase-PCR assay in patients with node-negative breast cancer not receiving adjuvant systemic therapy. Clin Cancer Res 11:3315–3319

Fan C, Oh DS, Wessels L et al (2006) Concordance among gene-expression-based predictors for breast cancer. N Engl J Med 355:560–569

Filipits M, Rudas M, Jakesz R et al (2011) A new molecular predictor of distant recurrence in ER-positive, HER2-negative breast cancer adds independent information to conventional clinical risk factors. Clin Cancer Res 17:6012–6020

Fisher B, Dignam J, Bryant J et al (1996) Five versus more than five years of tamoxifen therapy for breast cancer patients with negative lymph nodes and estrogen receptor-positive tumors. J Natl Cancer Inst 88:1529–1542

Fisher B, Dignam J, Wolmark N et al (1999) Tamoxifen in treatment of intraductal breast cancer: national surgical adjuvant breast and bowel project B-24 randomised controlled trial. Lancet 353:1993–2000

Fisher B, Jeong J, Dignam J et al (2001a) Findings from recent national surgical adjuvant breast and bowel project adjuvant studies in stage I breast cancer. J Natl Cancer Inst Monogr 30:62–66

Fisher B, Dignam J, Bryant J, Wolmark N (2001b) Five versus more than five years of tamoxifen for lymph node-negative breast cancer: updated findings from the National Surgical Adjuvant Breast and Bowel Project B-14 randomized trial. J Natl Cancer Inst 93:684–690

Foekens JA, Atkins D, Zhang Y et al (2006) Multicenter validation of a gene expression-based prognostic signature in lymph node-negative primary breast cancer. J Clin Oncol 24(11):1665–1671

Gianni L, Zambetti M, Clark K et al (2005) Gene expression profiles in paraffin-embedded core biopsy tissue predict response to chemotherapy in women with locally advanced breast cancer. J Clin Oncol 23:7265–7277

Glas AM, Floore A, Delahaye LJ et al (2006) Converting a breast cancer microarray signature into a high-throughput diagnostic test. BMC Genomics 7:278

Goetz M, Suman V, Ingle JN et al (2006) A two gene expression ratio of HOXB13 and IL-17BR for prediction of recurrence and survival in women receiving adjuvant tamoxifen. Clin Cancer Res 12:2080–2087

Goldhirsch A, Glick JH, Gelber RD et al (2001) Meeting highlights: international consensus panel on the treatment of primary breast cancer. seventh international conference on adjuvant therapy of primary breast cancer. J ClinOncol 19(18):3817–3827

Goldhirsch A, Glick JH, Gelber RD et al (2005) Meeting highlights: international expert consensus on the primary therapy of early breast cancer 2005. Ann Oncol 16(10):1569–1583

Goldhirsch A, Ingle JN, Gelber RD et al (2009) Thresholds for therapies: highlights of the St Gallen international expert consensus on the primary therapy of early breast cancer 2009. Ann Oncol 20:1319–1329

Goldstein LJ, Gray R, Badve S et al (2008) Prognostic utility of the 21-gene assay in hormone receptor-positive operable breast cancer compared with classical clinicopathologic features. J Clin Oncol 26:4063–4071

Habel LA, Shak S, Jacobs MK et al (2006) A population-based study of tumor gene expression and risk of breast cancer death among lymph node-negative patients. Breast Cancer Res 8:R25

Harris L, Fritsche H, Mennel R et al (2007) American society of clinical oncology 2007 update of recommendations for the use of tumor markers in breast cancer. J Clin Oncol 25:5287–5312

Henry L, Stojadinovic A, Swain S et al (2009) The influence of a gene expression profile on breast cancer decisions. J Surg Oncol 99:319–323

Hornberger J, Chien R (2010) Meta-analysis of the decision impact of the 21-gene breast cancer recurrence score in clinical practice. San Antonio breast cancer symposium 2010. Abstract-20609

Hornberger JC, Chjien R (2011) Meta-analysis of the decision impact of the 21-gene breast cancer recurrence score in clinical practice. Presented at the 2011 St. Gallen oncology conference. St. Gallen, Switzerland, 2011

Hughes LL, Wang M, Page DL et al (2009) Local excision alone without irradiation for ductal carcinoma in situ of the breast: a trial of the Eastern cooperative oncology group. J Clin Oncol 27 (32):5319–5324

Ivshina AC, George J, Senko O et al (2006) Genetic reclassification of histologic grade delineates new clinical subtypes of breast cancer. Cancer Res 66:10292–10301

Jankowitz R, Chivukula M, Ma XJ et al (2010) Predictive value of the Theros Breast Cancer Index (TBCI) for distant recurrence and overall survival (OS) in comparison to Adjuvant! Online and clinicopathologic characteristics in women with lymph node (LN)-negative, ER-positive breast cancer (BCa). J ClinOncol 28(suppl.):15s abstr 10582

Jansen MPHM, Sieuwerts AM, Look MP et al (2007) HOXB13-to-IL17BR expression ratio is related with tumor aggressiveness and response to tamoxifen of recurrent breast cancer: a retrospective study. J Clin Oncol 25:662–668

Jerevall PL, Brommesson S, Strand C et al (2008) Exploring the two-gene ratio in breast cancer-independent roles for HOXB13 and IL17BR in prediction of clinical outcome. Breast Cancer Res Treat 107:225–234

Joensuu H, Pylkkanen L, Toikkanen S (1998) Long-term survival in node-positive breast cancer treated by locoregional therapy alone. Br J Cancer 78(6):795–799

Klang S, Hammerman A, Liebermann N et al (2010) Economic implications of 21-gene breast cancer risk assay from the perspective of an Israeli managed healthcare organization. Value Health 13 (381):387

Knauer M, Mook S, Rutgers EJ et al (2010) The predictive value of the 70-gene signature for adjuvant chemotherapy in early breast cancer. Breast Cancer Res Treat 120(3):655–661

Liang H, Brufsky AM, Lembersky BB et al (2007) A retrospective analysis of the impact of oncotype DX low recurrence score results on treatment decisions in a single academic breast cancer center. Breast Cancer Res Treat 106:S105 [Abstract 2061]

Liedtke C, Hatzis C, Symmans WF et al (2009) Genomic grade index is associated with response to chemotherapy in patients with breast cancer. J Clin Oncol 27(19):3185–3191

Lo SS, Mumby PB, Norton J et al (2010) Prospective multicenter study of the impact of the 21-gene recurrence score assay on medical oncologist and patient adjuvant breast cancer treatment selection. J ClinOncol 28:1671–1676

Loi S, Haibe-Kains B, Desmedt C et al (2007) Definition of clinically distinct molecular subtypes in estrogen receptor-positive breast carcinomas through genomic grade. J Clin Oncol 25:1239–1246

Ma XJ, Wang Z, Ryan PD et al (2004) A two-gene expression ratio predicts clinical outcome in breast cancer patients treated with tamoxifen. Cancer Cell 5:607–616

Ma XJ, Hilsenbeck SG, Wang W et al (2006) The HOXB13:IL17BR expression index is a prognostic factor in early-stage breast cancer. J Clin Oncol 24:4611–4619

Ma XJ, Salunga R, Dahiya S et al (2008) A five-gene molecular grade index and HOXB13:IL17BR are complementary prognostic factors in early stage breast cancer. Clin Cancer Res 14(9):2601–2608

Mamounas EP, Tang G, Fisher B et al (2010) Association between the 21-gene recurrence score assay and risk of locoregional recurrence in node-negative, estrogen receptor-positive breast cancer: results from NSABP B-14 and NSABP B-20. J Clin Oncol 28:1677–1683

Mook S, Schmidt MK, Viale G et al (2009) The 70-gene prognosis-signature predicts disease outcome in breast cancer patients with 1–3 positive lymph nodes in an independent validation study. Breast Cancer Res Treat 116:295–302

Mook S, Schmidt MK, Weigelt B et al (2010) The 70-gene prognosis signature predicts early metastasis in breast cancer patients between 55 and 70 years of age. Ann Oncol 21:717–722

National Institutes of Health (2000) Adjuvant therapy for breast cancer. NIH Consens Statement Online 17:1–23

NCCN clinical practice guidelines in oncology: breast cancer version 2.2011. Available at http://www.nccn.org/professionals/physician_gls/pdf/breast.pdf. Accessed December 2011

Nielsen TO, Parker JS, Leung S et al (2010) A comparison of PAM50 intrinsic subtyping with immunohistochemistry and clinical prognostic factors in tamoxifen-treated estrogen receptor–positive breast cancer. Clin Cancer Res 16:5222–5232

Olivotto IA, Bajdik CD, Ravdin PM et al (2005) Population based validation of the prognostic model ADJUVANT! for early breast cancer. J Clin Oncol 23:2716–2725

Oratz R, Paul D, Cohn A, Sedlacek S (2007) Impact of a commercial reference laboratory test Recurrence Score on decision making in early-stage breast cancer. J Oncol Pract 3:182–186

Page DL (1991) Prognosis and breast cancer recognition of lethal and favorable prognostic types. Am J SurgPathol 15(4):334–349

Paik S, Shak S, Tang G, et al (2003) Multi-gene RT-PCR assay for predicting recurrence in node negative breast cancer patients – NSABP studies B-20 and B-14 [abstract].Breast Cancer Res Treat 82:A16. (http://www.sabcs.org)

Paik S, Shak S, Tang G et al (2004a) A multigene assay to predict recurrence of tamoxifen-treated, node-negative breast cancer. N Engl J Med 351:2817–2826

Paik S, Shak S, Tang G et al (2004b) Expression of the 21 genes in the recurrence score assay and prediction of the clinical benefit from tamoxifen in NSABP study B-14 and chemotherapy in NSABP study B-20. Br Ca Res Treat 88:S15 abstr 24

Paik S, Shak S, Tang G (2005) Risk classification of breast cancer patients by the recurrence score assay: comparison to guidelines based on patient age, tumor size, and tumor grade. Poster presented at the 28th Annual San Antonio Breast Cancer Symposium, San Antonio, Texas, 2005

Paik S, Tang G, Shak S et al (2006) Gene expression and benefit of chemotherapy in women with node-negative, estrogen receptor-positive breast cancer. J Clin Oncol 24:3726–3734

Parker JS, Mullins M, Maggie CU et al (2009) Supervised Risk Predictor of Breast Cancer Based on Intrinsic Subtypes. J Clin Oncol 27:1160–1167

Perou CM, Sorlie T, Eisen MB et al (2000) Molecular portraits of human breast tumours. Nature 406(6797):747–752

Pusztai L, Hatzis C, Cardoso F et al (2008) Combined use of genomic prognostic and treatment response predictors in lymph node-negative breast cancer. J Clin Oncol 26:2008 (May 20 suppl; abstr 527)

Ravdin PM, Siminoff LA, Davis GJ et al (2001) Computer program to assist in making decisions about adjuvant therapy for women with early breast cancer. J ClinOncol 19(4):980–991

Reid JF, Lusa L, De Cecco L et al (2005) Limits of predictive models using microarray data for breast cancer clinical treatment outcome. J Natl Cancer Inst 97:927–930

Reis-Filho JS, Pusztai L (2011) Gene expression profiling in breast cancer: classification, prognostication, and prediction. Lancet 378:1812–1823

Reyal F, van Vliet MH, Armstrong NJ et al (2008) A comprehensive analysis of prognostic signatures reveals the high predictive capacity of the proliferation, immune response and RNA splicing modules in breast cancer. Breast Cancer Res 10:R93

Ring BZ, Seitz RS, Beck R et al (2006) Novel prognostic immuno-histochemical biomarker panel for estrogen receptor-positive breast cancer. J Clin Oncol 24:3039–3047

Rosen PP, Groshen S, Saigo PE et al (1989) Pathological prognostic factors in stage I (T1N0M0) and stage II (T1N1M0) breast carcinoma: a study of 644 patients with median follow-up of 18 years. J ClinOncol 7(9):1239–1251

Ross DT, Kim C-Y, Tang G et al (2008) Chemosensitivity and stratification by a five monoclonal antibody immunohistochemistry test in the NSABP B14 and B20 trials. Clin Cancer Res 14:6602–6609

Solin LJ, Gray R, Baehner FL, et al (2011) A quantitative multigene RT-PCR assay for predicting recurrence risk after surgical excision alone without irradiation for ductal carcinoma in situ (DCIS): a prospective validation study of the DCIS score from ECOG E5194. San Antonio breast cancer symposium 2011, abstract # S4-6

Sotiriou C, Wirapati P, Loi S et al (2006) Gene expression profiling in breast cancer: understanding the molecular basis of histologic grade to improve prognosis. J Natl Cancer Inst 98:262–272

Straver ME, Glas AM, Hannemann J et al (2010) The 70-gene signature as a response predictor for neoadjuvant chemotherapy in breast cancer. Breast Cancer Res Treat 119:551–558

Tang G, Cuzick J, Wale C et al (2010) Recurrence risk of node-negative and ER-positive early-stage breast cancer patients by combining recurrence score, pathologic, and clinical information: a meta-analysis approach. J Clin Oncol 28(Suppl):abstr 509

Tang G, Shak S, Paik S et al (2011a) Comparison of the prognostic and predictive utilities of the 21-gene recurrence score assay and adjuvant! for women with node-negative, estrogen receptor-positive breast cancer: results from NSABP B-14 and NSABP B-20. Breast Cancer Res Treat 127:133–142

Tang G, Cuzick J, Constantino JP et al (2011b) Risk of recurrence and chemotherapy benefit for patients with node-negative, estrogen receptor-positive breast cancer: recurrence Score alone and integrated with pathologic and clinical factors. J Clin Oncol 29:4365–4372

Thanasoulis T, Brown A, Frazier T (2008) The role of Oncotype DX assay on appropriate treatment for estrogen positive, lymph node negative invasive breast cancer. American Society of Breast Surgeons Annual Meeting, New York, 2008

Toussaint J, Sieuwerts AM, Haibe-Kains B et al (2009) Improvement of the clinical applicability of the Genomic Grade Index through a qRT-PCR test performed on frozen and formalin-fixed paraffin-embedded tissues. BMC Genomics 10:424

van de Vijver MJ, He YD, van't Veer LJ et al (2002) A gene-expression signature as a predictor of survival in breast cancer. N Engl J Med 347:1999–2009

van't Veer LJ, Dai H, van de Vijver MJ et al (2002) Gene expression profiling predicts clinical outcome of breast cancer. Nature 415 (530):536

Wang Y, Klijn JG, Zhang Y et al (2005) Gene-expression profiles to predict distant metastasis of lymph-node-negative primary breast cancer. Lancet 365:671

Weigelt B, Horlings HM, Kreike B et al (2008) Refinement of breast cancer classification by molecular characterization of histological special types. J Pathol 216:141–150

Wirapati P, Sotiriou C, Kunkel S et al (2008) Meta-analysis of gene expression profiles in breast cancer: toward a unified understanding of breast cancer subtyping and prognosis signatures. Breast Cancer Res 10:R65

Wittner BS, Sgroi DC, Ryan PD et al (2008) Analysis of the MammaPrint breast cancer assay in a predominantly postmeno-pausal cohort. Clin Cancer Res 14:2988–2993

Biology of DCIS and Progression to Invasive Disease

Sanaz A. Jansen

Contents

Abstract

Ductal carcinoma in situ (DCIS) is a non-invasive breast cancer in which neoplastic cells are confined within the breast milk duct basement membrane. Prior to the widespread use of screening mammography DCIS was a rare diagnosis, but now comprises 20–30 % of all newly diagnosed breast cancers in the US. This diagnosis is often treated in a fashion similar to invasive breast cancer. Standard treatment typically consists of breast-conserving surgery (with or without radiotherapy) or mastectomy. There is a growing clinical concern that many patients with DCIS are being over-treated since their disease will never progress to invasive life-threatening carcinomas. But how can this indolent subset be identified? A better understanding of the biology of DCIS and how it transforms into invasive cancer will shed light on this important clinical goal. In this chapter, we identify important molecular pathways responsible for regulating cellular proliferation, apoptosis, and genome integrity that are altered in DCIS. We find surprisingly few differences on a genomic or gene-expression level between DCIS and invasive disease. We introduce diverse models of DCIS progression that are stochastic versus predetermined and discuss how the empirical data supports or challenges these models. Due to the considerable difficulty of studying DCIS, many unanswered questions remain. Improvements in molecular assays and model systems may provide further insights into the etiology and natural history of this disease entity.

S. A. Jansen (✉)
Mouse Cancer Genetics Program, National Cancer Institute,
Frederick National Laboratory for Cancer Research,
1050 Boyles Street, Building 560 Rm 32-24,
Frederick, MD 21702, USA
e-mail: jansensa@mail.nih.gov

Abbreviations

DCIS	Ductal carcinoma in situ
DNA	Deoxyribonucleic acid
ER	Estrogen receptor
FISH	Fluorescence in situ hybridization

J. Strauss et al. (eds.), *Breast Cancer Biology for the Radiation Oncologist*, Medical Radiology. Radiation Oncology,
DOI: 10.1007/174_2012_647, © Springer-Verlag Berlin Heidelberg 2012
Published Online: 19 June 2012

GEM   Genetically engineered mice
HER2   Human epidermal growth factor receptor 2
IDC   Invasive ductal carcinoma
IHC   Immunohistochemistry
MIN   Mammary intraepithelial neoplasia
MRI   Magnetic resonance imaging
PR   Progesterone receptor
RNA   Ribonucleic acid
TDLU   Terminal ductal lobular unit

1   What is Ductal Carcinoma In Situ?

The human breast is composed of thousands of terminal ductal lobular units (TDLUs), clusters of glands that produce milk that is carried to the nipple via a coalescing network of milk ducts (Sgroi 2010). A cross-section through this mammary ductal system reveals an inner layer of luminal epithelial cells, myoepithelial cells, and a basement membrane (Fig. 1). Ductal carcinoma in situ (DCIS) is a non-invasive breast cancer, arising primarily in the TDLUs (Wellings et al. 1975), where the proliferating neoplastic cells are still confined within the basement membrane (Allred 2010). DCIS is thought to be a non-obligate precursor to the most common invasive breast cancer, invasive ductal carcinoma (IDC), wherein cancerous cells have invaded beyond the basement membrane into the surrounding breast stroma (Fig. 1).

Before the widespread use of screening mammography, DCIS comprised only ~1–2 % of all newly diagnosed breast cancers (Allred 2010). These DCIS lesions were large, palpable, and described as "comedo" due to the necrotic ooze that poured out of them when squeezed. With the advent of screening mammography, the incidence of DCIS skyrocketed to comprising 20–30 % of newly diagnosed breast cancers in the US today (Kerlikowske 2010; Virnig et al. 2010). Mammographic screening also revealed a previously unexplored spectrum of DCIS lesions with diverse histological, molecular, and genetic characteristics. In this chapter, we will delve into what is known regarding the biology of this remarkably heterogeneous disease, and how it transforms itself into invasive carcinomas.

Radiographically, the classic presentation of DCIS comes in the form of calcifications on X-ray mammography, with a diversity of shapes and spatial distributions (D'Orsi 2010). Magnetic resonance imaging (MRI), while not as widely used X-ray mammography, has the highest sensitivity for DCIS of all clinically used imaging modalities (Kuhl et al. 2007). DCIS presents with a distinctive nonmass-like morphology on MRI, with clumped internal enhancement in a segmental, linear, or regional distribution (Jansen et al. 2007; Lehman 2010; Jansen 2011). Although DCIS is a preinvasive cancer, it is not necessarily small—the average size of DCIS is 10–20 mm (Allegra et al. 2010), but some lesions can extend through most of a major breast lobe (Tot 2010).

Histologically, DCIS is classified according to metrics initially developed for IDC such as grade. DCIS is categorized as low, intermediate, or high grade based on a variety of nuclear features including size and mitotic activity. Overall, DCIS lesions are classified either as well-, moderately-, or poorly-differentiated depending on how closely they resemble normal cells (Fig. 1) (Allred 2010). Unlike IDC, DCIS has distinctive growth/architectural patterns describing how the cells are distributed within the duct lumen: solid, papillary, micropapillary, cribriform or comedo. Necrosis is extensive and predominant in comedo DCIS while focal or absent in the other architectural subtypes.

Current treatment paradigms for DCIS include mastectomy (Hwang 2010), lumpectomy alone, or lumpectomy with radiation therapy (Kane et al. 2010). Approximately 20 % of DCIS patients treated with lumpectomy alone experience a recurrence, half as DCIS and half as invasive cancer (Kerlikowske et al. 2010). Both radiation therapy and adjuvant Tamoxifen have been shown to reduce recurrence rates by approximately 50 % in DCIS (Correa et al. 2010; Eng-Wong et al. 2010; Solin 2010). Given current management strategies, the prognosis for DCIS is excellent with a 10-year disease-specific survival rates of 98 % (Bijker and van Tienhoven 2010; Kerlikowske et al. 2010; Schnitt 2010). Concomitantly high incidence and survival rates imply that by 2020, an estimated 1 million women will be living with a diagnosis of DCIS in the US alone (Allegra et al. 2010).

In many ways, DCIS represents a success story in breast cancer management—the combination of early detection and effective treatments yields excellent cure rates in these patients. However, there is a growing clinical concern that a significant portion of DCIS patients are actually being *over*-diagnosed and *over*-treated, as indirect evidence suggests that approximately 50 % of DCIS will not progress to invasive, life-threatening diseases (Erbas et al. 2006; Kuerer et al. 2009; Allegra et al. 2010). However, there is no way now to identify this subset of women with indolent disease who may benefit from less aggressive therapeutic interventions. As highlighted by a 2009 National Institutes of Health State of the Science Conference Statement, the primary task for research going forward is to identify subsets of DCIS patients based on their risk of progression to invasive carcinoma (Allegra et al. 2010). An important step toward achieving this goal is to better characterize the biology of DCIS and understand the key events responsible for its transition to invasive carcinoma.

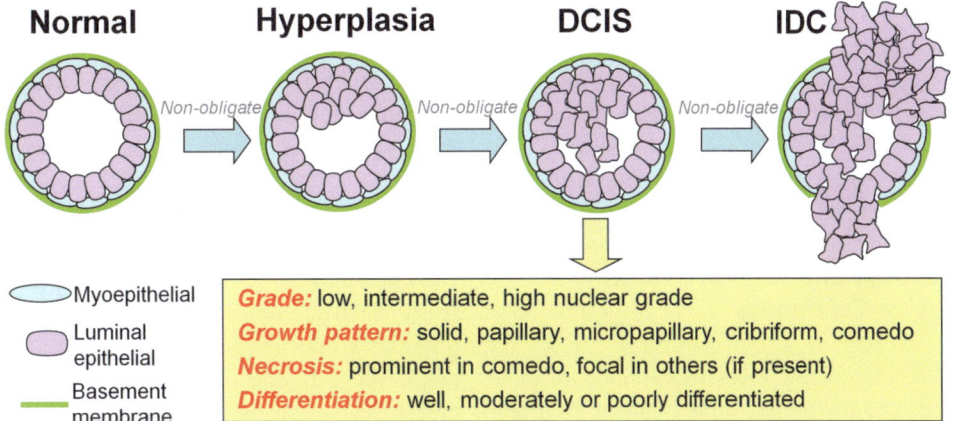

Fig. 1 The stages of breast cancer. Within the normal mammary duct and TDLU, an inner layer of luminal epithelial cells and a basal layer of myoepithelial cells are surrounded by a basement membrane. In benign hyperplasia, epithelial cells have proliferated within the duct while retaining a largely normal phenotype. In ductal carcinoma in situ (DCIS), the cells appear phenotypically different from normal epithelia—poorly differentiated DCIS more so than well-differentiated DCIS—yet are still confined by the basement membrane. DCIS is classified into several subtypes based on its histopathological presentation, including grade, growth pattern, and necrosis. Once the neoplastic cells invade beyond a degraded basement membrane into the surrounding breast stroma, they have transitioned to invasive ductal carcinoma (IDC). In subsequent figures, the luminal cells, myoepithelial cells, and basement membranes are displayed with the same color scheme as shown above

2   The Biology of DCIS

Cancer is a genetic disease wherein malignant transformation is driven by changes in DNA. There are many types of alterations that can occur, including gross chromosomal gains/losses, genomic amplification, genomic rearrangements, activation of oncogenes, and inactivation of tumor suppressor genes via mutation, deletion, methylation, or transcriptional repression. As a consequence of these genomic events, the cancer transcriptome can exhibit marked irregularities compared to normal tissue. These transcriptional changes, usually represented by up or downregulated gene signatures in gene-expression profiles, are then translated into the proteome, resulting in proteins that are overexpressed, lost, or have amino-acid substitutions that confer gain or loss of function. Additionally, post-transcriptional and post-translational modifications not reflected at the mRNA level can also affect the function, stability, and distribution of proteins. Characterization of cancer at all levels—DNA, RNA, and protein—is a major goal of cancer biology, as it can elucidate both the molecular *pathways* critical for cancer etiology and identify *subtypes* of disease that provide prognostic information or predict therapeutic efficacy. For example, breast cancers that express estrogen receptor (ER) are often treated with selective ER modulators in an adjuvant setting.

In the larger context of breast cancer biology and evolution, DCIS is thought to be a precursor to IDC. However, it is not direct observation of DCIS progression to invasive disease in women that underpins this belief—due to the obligate surgical excision of newly diagnosed cancers including DCIS it is very challenging to track the natural history of disease in women (Erbas et al. 2006). Rather, the status of DCIS as a precursor to IDC is due to a large body of compelling yet indirect evidence demonstrating connections between the two. This evidence includes sharing similar risk factors (Kerlikowske 2010), the increased risk of recurrence as IDC at the tumor bed for women with DCIS, frequent co-existence of DCIS and IDC together in the same lesion (Allred et al. 2008), and the finding that DCIS and IDC harbor many of the same molecular and genetic abnormalities (Polyak 2010). Further evidence temporally linking DCIS to IDC comes from follow-up of women with DCIS initially misdiagnosed as benign disease showing that 14–50 % eventually develop IDC (Erbas et al. 2006), and work in animal models where more direct observations of preneoplastic progression are possible (Maglione et al. 2001, 2004; Namba et al. 2004, 2006; Damonte et al. 2008). Although our primary focus is on DCIS, we will begin with a brief examination of the key biological features of invasive cancers. This will serve as a platform for our subsequent discussion of the genomic, gene-expression, and protein level characteristics of DCIS.

There is a caveat to what is presented below relating to the challenge of applying molecular assays to DCIS surgical specimens. Limitations include small patient cohorts, mixed screening and unscreened populations, and small lesion size. An additional challenge is getting access to tissue in the first place, particularly for patients with pure DCIS where most of the tissue must be processed to histologically rule out microscopic regions of invasion. Consequently, many studies describing the molecular features of DCIS often include lesions that have both IDC and DCIS components. The unavoidable limitations of studies of DCIS are important to consider when interpreting the empirical data.

2.1 The Genome and Transcriptome of Invasive Carcinoma

On the genomic level, grade I invasive carcinomas show low levels of genomic instability, with frequent recurrent loss of 16q and gain at 1q. Conversely, grade III invasive cancers show higher levels of genomic instability with amplification of 17q12, 11q13, loss of 8p, 11q, 13q, and gains of 1q, 8q, 17q, and 20q (Buerger et al. 1999a, b; Roylance et al. 1999). Grade II IDC can exhibit mixed features between these two (Sgroi 2010). The frequent loss of 16q in low but not high-grade carcinomas is salient for modeling breast cancer evolution. It suggests that the majority of grade III invasive carcinomas do not arise from a grade I precursor, as this would imply the recovery of genetic material at 16q. Rather, the restriction of the loss of 16q to low-grade invasive carcinoma suggests that the different grades of invasive carcinoma arise from different pathways. Empirical data complicate this interpretation since approximately 20 % of grade III IDC also harbor loss of 16q (Roylance et al. 1999), suggesting that the low to high-grade transition may occur in a subset of women. These high-grade lesions with loss of 16q are mostly ER+ (Smart et al. 2011).

Comprehensive gene expression profiling based on the influential studies by Perou et al. (2000) and Sorlie et al. (2001) have resulted in the molecular subtype classification of breast cancers into four categories. The major distinction is at the level of ER, and secondarily on the level of human epidermal growth factor receptor 2 (HER2). Two subtypes are ER–: the *basal* (HER2–) and *ERBB2* (HER2+) groups, and two subtypes are ER+: the *luminal A* (HER2–) and *luminal B* (HER2+) groups. These transcriptome-based subtypes correlate well with other histological and clinical features; luminal A and B often exhibit lower grade and more favorable prognosis compared to the basal and ERBB2 subtypes, which are often higher grade with poorer prognosis (Sorlie et al. 2001).

2.2 The Genome and Transcriptome of DCIS

Remarkably, there are essentially no progression-specific changes in DCIS compared to IDC on the genome or transcriptome level. On the contrary, the characteristics of DCIS mirror those of invasive breast cancer, including exhibiting distinct molecular characteristics by grade (Porter et al. 2001, 2003). Low-grade DCIS also harbors frequent recurrent loss of 16q, while high-grade DCIS shows a more complex genomic pattern with loss at 8p, 11q, 14q, gains at 1q, 8q, and 17q and high level of amplification at 17q12 and 11q13 (Buerger et al. 1999a, b; Hwang et al. 2004; Vincent-Salomon et al. 2008). DCIS can also be classified into the four molecular subtypes of breast cancer (basal, ERBB2, luminal A and B) that in turn correlate with different grades (Vincent-Salomon et al. 2008). This evidence suggests that the bulk of genetic transformation in breast cancer does not occur during the (putative) DCIS to IDC phase change. Indeed, Ma et al. performed gene-expression profiling comparisons of normal breast tissue, DCIS, and IDC lesions and found that the largest transcriptional changes occur from the normal to DCIS transition, not the DCIS to invasive transition (Ma et al. 2003). With these qualitative similarities between DCIS and IDC noted, it is important to point out that quantitative analysis does reveal differences, for example in the levels of gene expression (Ma et al. 2003) and in the proportions of molecular subtypes found (Vincent-Salomon et al. 2008; Clark et al. 2011; Yu et al. 2011). Therefore, while similar genes may be affected in DCIS versus IDC, there may be differences in the dynamics (i.e., timing and levels) of such transcription.

Thus, from a genome and transcriptome perspective, we have not found molecular alterations that are specific to DCIS and not invasive disease. Rather there are dramatic changes from normal tissue to DCIS, and also between different grades regardless of whether invasive or noninvasive (Ma et al. 2003). This evidence further supports a multi-pathway grade-specific model of breast cancer progression that extends to the preinvasive stage.

2.3 Molecular Markers of DCIS

Analysis of protein expression in DCIS, most often assessed via immunohistochemistry (IHC) on tissue sections, is an important tool for studying the molecular pathways altered in DCIS and identifying subtypes of disease based on differential protein expression. An advantage of IHC is that the spatial distribution of proteins, both within the cell (i.e., cytoplasmic or nuclear) and across the lesion, can be visualized. An inherent limitation is that for many molecular markers, methods for determining positivity in DCIS have not been fully standardized. Most commonly, a lesion is classified as positive ('+') if a certain threshold number of cells within the lesion exhibit positive staining, and negative ('−') if that threshold is not met (Lari and Kuerer 2011). The most studied molecular markers in DCIS are ER

Table 1 Summary of the molecular markers used to characterize DCIS

Molecular markers	Functions	Molecular signatures correlating with increased risk of recurrence
ER, PR	Steroid receptors	ER−
HER2	Regulates proliferation and apoptosis	HER2+ ER−/HER2+ ER−/HER2 +/Ki-67+
p53	Regulates cell-cycle, apoptosis, and genomic stability; p53 is an important tumor suppressor	p53+
Rb/p16 pathway	Regulates cell-cycle; Rb is an important tumor suppressor	p16+
Ki-67	Proliferation marker	Ki-67+
COX-2	Enzyme for prostaglandin synthesis; expressed during inflammatory response	COX-2+ p16+/COX-2-/Ki-67+ (DCIS recurrence) p16+/COX-2+/Ki-67+ (invasive recurrence)
Akt/PTEN pathway	Regulates proliferation, survival and motility; PTEN is an important tumor suppressor	
BRCA1/2	DNA damage repair	
c-myc	Transcription factor that can activate proliferation; c-myc is a proto-oncogene	
VEGF, vascular patterns	Angiogenesis and vascular markers	
Cyclin A, cyclin E, p21, p27	Cell-cycle regulators	p21+
Bcl-2, Bax, Survivin	Apoptosis regulators	Bcl-2− Survivin+

Included are the molecular signatures that have been shown to correlate with an increased risk of subsequent recurrence in some reports

and HER2. However, other important signaling pathways responsible for regulating proliferation, apoptosis, angiogenesis, and genome stability have also been examined (Lari and Kuerer 2011) (Table 1).

- *Estrogen and progesterone receptors.* Approximately 70–80 % of DCIS lesions are ER+ (Tamimi et al. 2008; Kerlikowske et al. 2010). ER+ DCIS is less likely to be high grade, HER2+, p53+, and Ki-67+ or display comedo growth patterns (Lari and Kuerer 2011). PR expression correlates closely with ER.
- *HER2.* HER2 is a member of the ErbB family of proteins and is involved in regulating cellular proliferation and apoptosis through a variety of signaling pathways, including MAPK, Akt, and STAT. Approximately 20–30 % of DCIS patients have HER2 overexpression (Tamimi et al. 2008; Kerlikowske et al. 2010), as assessed by IHC or fluorescence in situ hybridization (FISH) to measure amplification of the ErbB2 gene. HER2+ DCIS is more likely to be ER−, PR−, Bcl-2−, p53+, Ki-67+, p21+, have high nuclear grade and exhibit comedo necrosis (Lari and Kuerer 2011). Although the proportion of HER2+ DCIS is comparable to IDC, the triple-negative i.e., ER−/PR−/HER2− phenotype is less common in DCIS (Kuerer et al. 2009)
- *p53.* p53 is an important tumor suppressor protein that plays a critical role in a cell-cycle regulation, apoptosis, and genomic stability. Mutations in the TP53 gene occur

in approximately 20 % of invasive breast cancers and 10–30 % of DCIS (Livasy et al. 2007; Kerlikowske et al. 2010) and can manifest itself on IHC as accumulated p53 protein expression. DCIS lesions that are p53+ are more likely to have high nuclear grade and comedo necrosis (Lari and Kuerer 2011). Likewise, TP53 mutations are more frequently observed in basal-like and HER2+ DCIS than those in the luminal group (Polyak 2010). As discussed in more detail below, p53 expression is correlated with increased intratumor heterogeneity in DCIS, which may arise as a result of increased genomic instability upon aberrant p53 activity.

- *Rb/p16 pathway.* A key regulator of cellular proliferation is the Rb tumor suppressor pathway. Rb functions to inhibit expression of genes required for cellular proliferation by assembling transcription repression complexes. This activity is reduced in proliferating cells by the action of CDK/cyclin complexes that phosphorylate Rb. In particular, the CDK4/cyclin D complex is the rate-limiting step for Rb inactivation; this complex is itself counteracted by p16. The Rb-cyclinD-p16 network defines a pathway that is functionally inactivated in most cancers, although Rb itself may not be mutated or lost. For example, simultaneous expression of both p16 and Ki-67 could be indicative of Rb functional loss, as recently suggested by Witkiewicz et al. for DCIS

(Witkiewicz et al. 2011). Abrogation of the Rb pathway has recently been proposed as a mechanism by which DCIS can survive the hypoxic and stressful intraductal environment (Espina and Liotta 2011). Approximately 70, 60, and 35 % of DCIS lesions are Rb+, cyclin D1+, and p16+, respectively (Gauthier et al. 2007; Millar et al. 2007; Kulkarni et al. 2008; Okumura et al. 2008; Kerlikowske et al. 2010), while 22 % are both p16+/Ki-67+ (Kerlikowske et al. 2010).

• *Akt/PTEN pathway.* The Akt pathway regulates many diverse biological functions, including cellular motility, proliferation, and survival. Components of this pathway, particularly PTEN, are deregulated in a wide spectrum of human cancers. The PTEN tumor suppressor is an important negative regulator of the Akt pathway, and is altered in approximately 40 % of invasive breast cancers. Using tissue microarrays comprised of pure DCIS and IDC, Bose et al. evaluated the expression of Akt pathway members at different stages of breast cancer progression. They found that Akt and its downstream proteins mTor and S6 are activated in 30 % of DCIS and IDC lesions. Interestingly, PTEN was differentially expressed by stage: only 11 % of DCIS exhibited loss of PTEN compared to 26 % of invasive cancers (Bose et al. 2006). PTEN loss has also been linked to the basal subtype of DCIS (Polyak 2010).

• *BRCA1/2.* The tumor suppressors BRCA1 and BRCA2 function to repair damaged DNA. Women with deleterious mutations in the BRCA1/2 genes are at high risk for developing invasive breast cancers with earlier onset. A prior misconception had been that the natural history of BRCA-related tumorigenesis differed significantly from its sporadic counterpart, by passing very quickly through the in situ phase (if at all). However, more recent studies have reaffirmed DCIS as a relevant stage in BRCA-related breast cancer. In BRCA mutation carriers, DCIS is diagnosed in comparable proportion as in other patient cohorts (Hwang et al. 2007; Arun et al. 2009). Furthermore, the prevalence of BRCA1 and BRCA2 mutations among DCIS lesions is comparable to that of invasive carcinomas (Claus et al. 2005; Smith et al. 2007). Interestingly, recent evidence suggests that DCIS is more difficult to *detect* with MRI in BRCA1 mutation carriers compared to other high-risk women including BRCA2 mutation carriers (Sardanelli et al. 2010; Jansen 2011; Warner et al. 2011). This points to possible differences in underlying physical or physiological properties, leading to evasion of MRI detection.

• *c-myc.* The proto-oncogene c-myc is a transcription factor that plays a role in proliferation, malignant transformation, and apoptosis. The observed genomic alterations in DCIS implicate the activation of the c-myc gene located at 8q24; this includes frequent observation in DCIS of gains at 8q and the loss of CTCF, a transcriptional regulator of c-myc, at 16q. Approximately 60 % of DCIS are c-myc+, and these lesions are more likely to be HER2+ and proliferative (Altintas et al. 2009).

• *Angiogenesis.* As a non-invasive stage of breast cancer, DCIS is not necessarily associated with dense, leaky neovasculature as invasive cancers can be. In carefully examining the vascular distribution associated with DCIS, Guidi et al. found they could be categorized into two patterns: "diffusely" permeating blood vessels in the stroma, or vascular "cuffing" wherein blood vessels pack densely around neoplastic ducts (Guidi et al. 1994). Expression of VEGF, a potent angiogenic factor, has been found in approximately 85 % of DCIS lesions (Hieken et al. 2001).

• *Other markers.* Other important molecular markers including cell-cycle regulators, proliferation, and apoptosis markers have been found to be differentially expressed in subsets of DCIS. These include cyclin A, cyclin E, p21, p27, Bcl-2, Bax, Survivin, Ki-67, and COX-2 (Clark et al. 2011; Lari and Kuerer 2011). The latter two, used often to characterize invasive carcinomas, may be particularly relevant for DCIS. Ki-67 is a nuclear protein used as a cellular marker for proliferation. Approximately 40 % of DCIS lesions are positive for Ki-67 (Livasy et al. 2007; Kerlikowske et al. 2010). Increased Ki-67 expression is associated with high grade and comedo necrosis (Lari and Kuerer 2011). Alterations to COX-2 expression and the accumulation of its enzymatic product prostaglandins have been implicated in a variety of human cancers, including approximately 45–65 % of DCIS (Boland et al. 2004; Kerlikowske et al. 2010; Glover et al. 2011). COX-2 expression has been associated with high nuclear grade and the Ki-67+/ER− molecular signatures (Lari and Kuerer 2011).

In analyzing protein expression levels, we have identified key pathways governing proliferation, apoptosis, and genomic stability that are altered in DCIS, and have also revealed subtypes of DCIS wherein molecular markers are differentially expressed i.e., exhibit marked *inter*-tumor heterogeneity. However, DCIS also exhibits considerable *intra*-tumor heterogeneity as it is often possible to find a variety of grades and molecular subtypes within the same lesion (Polyak 2007). This heterogeneity could be explained by several possible mechanisms, including genomic instability due to telomere shortening, epigenetic instability, malignant stem cells, or phenotypic plasticity (Chin et al. 2004; Marusyk and Polyak 2010). In studying clonal diversity, Allred et al. observed that 50 % of DCIS lesions include diverse nuclear grades and molecular markers, and that this intratumor heterogeneity correlated with p53 expression on IHC (Allred et al. 2008). They proposed that aberrant p53 activity leads to genetic instability and the development of multiple neoplastic clones within the same lesion. These diverse regions in DCIS then compete for dominance, suggesting that poorly differentiated DCIS evolves from well-differentiated DCIS by randomly acquiring genetic defects. Intratumor heterogeneity itself may be a useful molecular marker for the potential of preinvasive cancers to progress to invasion—clonal diversity measures in Barret's esophagus can predict progression to esophageal adenocarcinoma (Maley et al. 2006)—although this has not been fully explored in DCIS. The mechanisms underlying the etiology of intratumor heterogeneity in DCIS are still poorly defined. They may be better understood within the context of models of preinvasive cancer progression.

3 Progression of DCIS to Invasive Disease

Until now we have mostly focused on a thorough molecular characterization of DCIS at the snapshot in time that it was diagnosed. But how does DCIS evolve over time and progress to invasive carcinoma? Investigating this question will not only shed light on the etiology of breast cancer, but will also address the critical clinical goal of identifying subsets of DCIS patients based on risk of progression to invasive carcinoma (Allegra et al. 2010). With this clinical motivation in mind, we will ask the following two questions of the DCIS progression models we present below: given a newly diagnosed DCIS lesion, can it (i) predict the type of invasive cancer that will arise? and (ii) determine the risk of progression to invasive cancer?

3.1 Predictive Markers of DCIS Progression

The empirical data regarding molecular attributes that can predict risk of DCIS progression to IDC are murky due to the tremendous challenge of performing such investigations in humans. Limitations include small population sizes, lack of long-term follow-up of outcome, and difficulty controlling for different treatments. Perhaps most constraining is the clinical necessity of surgical excision of DCIS instead of observation—this precludes following its natural history to truly determine which features of DCIS predict the risk of progression to invasive carcinoma. As a surrogate endpoint, recurrence is used to assess progression of disease in most studies (Kerlikowske et al. 2010; Lari and Kuerer 2011). Higher nuclear grade, comedo growth pattern, necrosis, and positive surgical margins are linked with increased rates of local recurrence in DCIS (Shamliyan et al. 2010). Additionally, there is some evidence implicating the following molecular markers as correlating with a subsequent recurrence event (Table 1): ER−, PR−, HER2+, Ki67+, cyclin D1−, p21+, p53+, BCL-2−, Survivin+ and possibly most convincingly, p16+ and COX-2+ (Lari and Kuerer 2011; Rakovitch et al. 2012). The largest study to date was performed by Kerlikowske et al. examining a diversity of molecular markers in 1162 women diagnosed with DCIS (Kerlikowske et al. 2010). They found that the molecular signature p16+/COX-2−/Ki-67+ was predictive of a subsequent DCIS but not invasive recurrence, while the p16+/COX-2+/Ki-67+ signature was predictive of a subsequent invasive recurrence. This establishes a role for COX-2 in promoting invasive potential of DCIS, and also implicates aberrant Rb pathway activity in the p16+/Ki-67+ signature (Gauthier et al. 2007; Witkiewicz et al. 2011). They also found the ER−/HER2+ and ER−/HER2+/Ki-67+ signatures to correlate with DCIS recurrence. Although there are many caveats in such studies, the empirical data suggests it is possible for distinct molecular signatures to predict risk of DCIS progression to invasive carcinoma. But is this possibility consistent with models of breast cancer evolution?

3.2 Models of DCIS Progression

The traditional sequential model of cancer progression that has been proposed for many tissue types (Vogelstein et al. 1988) posits that genetic and epigenetic modifications accumulate gradually over time, governing the transition from normal to in situ and then invasive carcinoma (Fig. 2). Consequently, at the time of DCIS diagnosis it would not be possible to predict either the risk of progression or the type of invasive cancer that could arise because the transforming biological events conferring invasion have likely not yet occurred. However, the similarities we have seen between DCIS and IDC on the genome and transcriptome level leaves little room for genetic events to dictate the transition from preinvasive to invasive disease. Rather, it suggests that the bulk of malignant transformation within the epithelial cells has already occurred by the DCIS stage.

One possible mechanism for this relates to the cancer stem cell hypothesis (Fig. 3). As suggested by Cardiff et al. and others, a precancer stem cell, capable of self-renewal and reestablishing a preinvasive cancer, could be the cell of origin for DCIS (Cardiff and Borowsky 2010). An initiating tumorigenic event occurring in a precancer stem cell would in turn generate an intrinsic subtype of cancer based on both the characteristics of the initiating event itself and the target precancer stem cell. The biology of the lesion including its potential for progression to IDC is thus 'pre-encoded' in its preinvasive state. In this way, the critical somatic mutations that determine the cell's fate have already occurred before the appearance of DCIS and do not change significantly with progression to IDC. Subsequent epigenetic or microenvironment effects can modulate the timing of progression (Cardiff and Borowsky 2010).

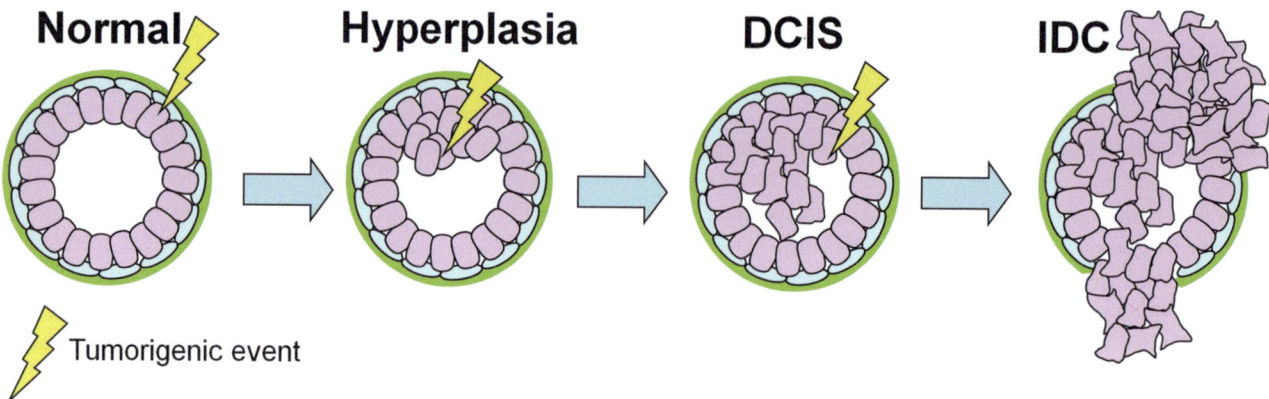

Fig. 2 The sequential model of DCIS progression. Tumorigenic events (e.g., oncogene activation, loss of tumor suppressor) targeting epithelial cells govern the transition between the different stages of breast cancer. In this model, an additional genetic hit is required for progression from DCIS to IDC. Therefore, at the time of DCIS diagnosis it is not possible to predict the type of invasive cancer that will arise

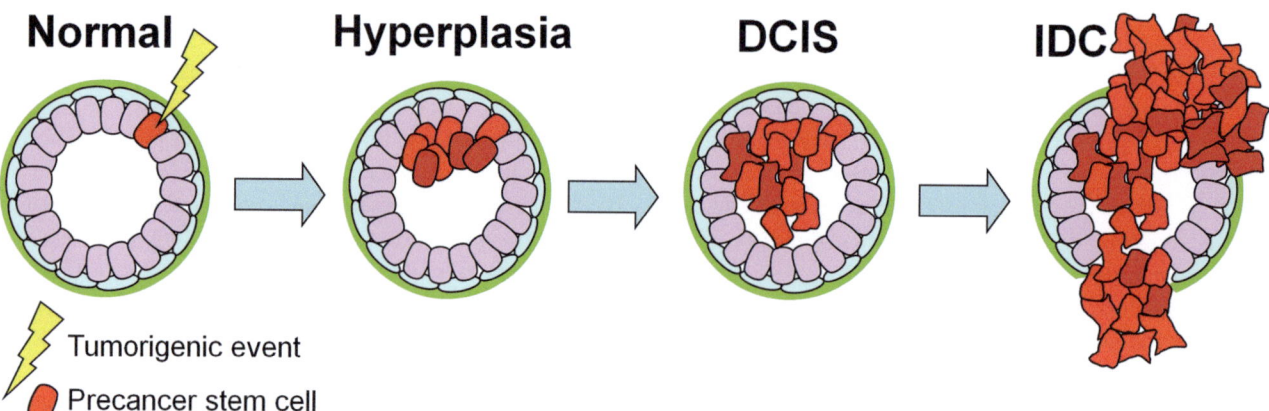

Fig. 3 The precancer stem cell model of DCIS progression. DCIS lesions arise as a result of tumorigenic events (e.g., oncogene activation, loss of tumor suppressor) occurring initially in a precancer stem cell. The molecular and biological properties of the ensuing DCIS lesion including its potential for progressing to invasive disease are pre-encoded within the initial target cell. In this way, the bulk of malignant transformation has occurred by the DCIS stage

An alternative mechanism is via the telomere crisis (Fig. 4) (Chin et al. 2004). Here, an initiating tumorigenic event, such as aberrant Rb activity, results in proliferation of epithelial cells leading to hyperplasia. However, because epithelial cells normally lack active telomerase, after extended proliferation the cells experience telomere shortening and eventually telomere loss. This telomere crisis leads to genomic instability and subsequent elimination by damage surveillance mechanisms. However, a few cells can reactivate telomerase, thereby surviving and continuing to clonally proliferate with stabilized genetic and epigenetic content. Continued low level instability can yield further evolution over time. Chin et al. position occurrence of the telomere crisis between hyperplasia and DCIS (Chin et al. 2004), suggesting that by the DCIS stage most genomic alterations have already occurred. Only one or two cells will survive the telomere crisis, and this post-transition immortal cell and its progeny would have a feature ascribed to tumor stem cells: active telomerase and the ability to propagate indefinitely.

It is therefore mechanistically conceivable via these two models that the majority of genetic and molecular events important for breast tumorigenesis have already occurred by the DCIS stage in epithelial cells. In both, genetic events occurring in a single cell of origin (either a precancer stem cell or the cell that survives the telomere crisis) largely define the molecular and biological path of the subsequent preinvasive and invasive cancer that will arise. Yet, the empirical data indicate there are not an infinite number of such paths; rather that only a few have been selected from an evolutionary perspective to lead to DCIS and IDC. There are four molecular subtypes of DCIS (basal, ErbB2, luminal A, luminal B), and three grades (low, intermediate, high). It has therefore

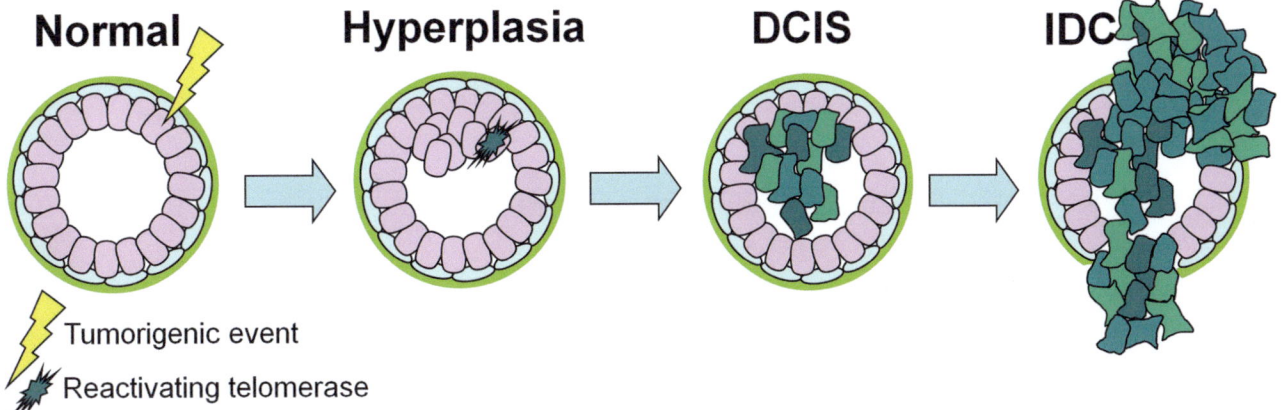

Fig. 4 The telomere crisis model of DCIS progression. An initiating proliferative event (e.g., loss of tumor suppressor) confers increased proliferation, such as aberrant Rb pathway activity. As the epithelial cells proliferate, their telomeres shorten and are eventually lost. This telomere crisis results in increased genomic instability and usually cell elimination due to damage surveillance mechanisms. However, a cell may survive beyond the crisis by reactivating telomerase. This cell then continues to clonally proliferate into DCIS, retaining the accrued genetic and epigenetic aberrations accumulated during the telomere crisis. In this way, the bulk of malignant transformation has occurred by the time a cell and its progeny become DCIS, and continued evolution is possible over time

been proposed that breast cancer progression occurs along grade and/or subtype specific pathways. While this would be consistent with the large-scale genomic similarities between DCIS and IDC, it does not account for the significant intra-tumor heterogeneity observed in DCIS. Allred et al. hypothesized that poorly differentiated DCIS can arise from well-differentiated DCIS as multiple clonal variants compete within the tumor in a process of clonal evolution and selection (Allred et al. 2008). Furthermore, the finding that a minority of high-grade ER+ invasive cancers also exhibit loss of 16q again supports the idea of low to high-grade progression in a subset of luminal breast cancers. In light of these observations, a modified version of the grade-specific pathway that accounts for the potential of low to high-grade progression in a subset of patients has been proposed (Fig. 5) (Sgroi 2010; Bombonati and Sgroi 2011).

Unlike the sequential model, in this multi-pathway grade-specific model it is possible to predict (at least to some extent) the type of invasive cancer that would subsequently arise if a newly diagnosed DCIS were left undisturbed. However, neither model provides compelling insight into whether a DCIS lesion is likely to progress in the first place. Perhaps this is because both narrowly focus on events occuring only within the tumor cells.

3.3 Role of the Microenvironment

Neoplastic epithelial cells exist within a complex micro-environment. The intraluminal microenvironment of DCIS consists of myoepithelial cells, inflammatory cells, and the basement membrane. Beyond the TDLU walls, the stromal microenvironment consists of fibroblasts, myofibroblasts, inflammatory cells, and endothelial cells. Given the paucity of tumor cell-specific genetic signatures of DCIS compared to IDC, recent efforts have shifted the spotlight from the biological events occurring within the neoplastic epithelial cell compartment to the microenvironment. Allinen et al. found significant differential gene expression in myofi-broblasts and myoepithelial cells of DCIS compared to normal ducts, including increased cathepsins F,K,L, MMP2, CXCL12, and CXCL14 (Allinen et al. 2004). Interestingly, they did not find significant genetic differences between these non-epithelial cells at different stages of progression, pointing to the possibility of epigenetic alterations in the microenvironment confirmed experimentally by Hu et al. (2005). Ma et al. performed global gene expression analysis of the epithelial versus stromal compartments in normal, DCIS, and IDC tissue. They found that over 300 genes were differentially regulated in the stromal compartment in DCIS versus IDC compared to only three epithelial genes. In particular, they implicate stroma produced MMPs (MMP2, MMP11, MMP14) as the key players in driving the DCIS to invasive transition (Ma et al. 2009). This evidence suggests that changes in the microenvironment transcriptome may condition DCIS lesions and affect whether and when they progress to an invasive cancer (Cardiff and Borowsky 2010). Conversely, clonally selected genetic alterations appear to be limited to the tumor cells (Allinen et al. 2004), although alternative theories suggest that a field of genetic instability can exist in the normal tissue around a tumor (Tot 2011).

Fig. 5 The multi-pathway, grade-specific model of DCIS progression. The evolution of cancer occurs along pathways determined largely by grade. Along the well-differentiated pathway, lesions are of low nuclear grade (*yellow cells*) with low-grade gene expression signatures (luminal A and B subtypes) and low genomic instability with frequent loss at 16q. In a minority of lesions, progression from low to intermediate (*green cells*) and high (*blue cells*) grade lesions is possible (*gray arrows*). Along the poorly differentiated pathway, lesions are of higher nuclear grade with high-grade gene expression profiles (basal and ERBB2 subtypes) and high genomic instability. Empirical data regarding the genomic and gene expression similarities between DCIS and IDC, as well as the intra-lesion heterogeneity in DCIS, can be consistent with this model

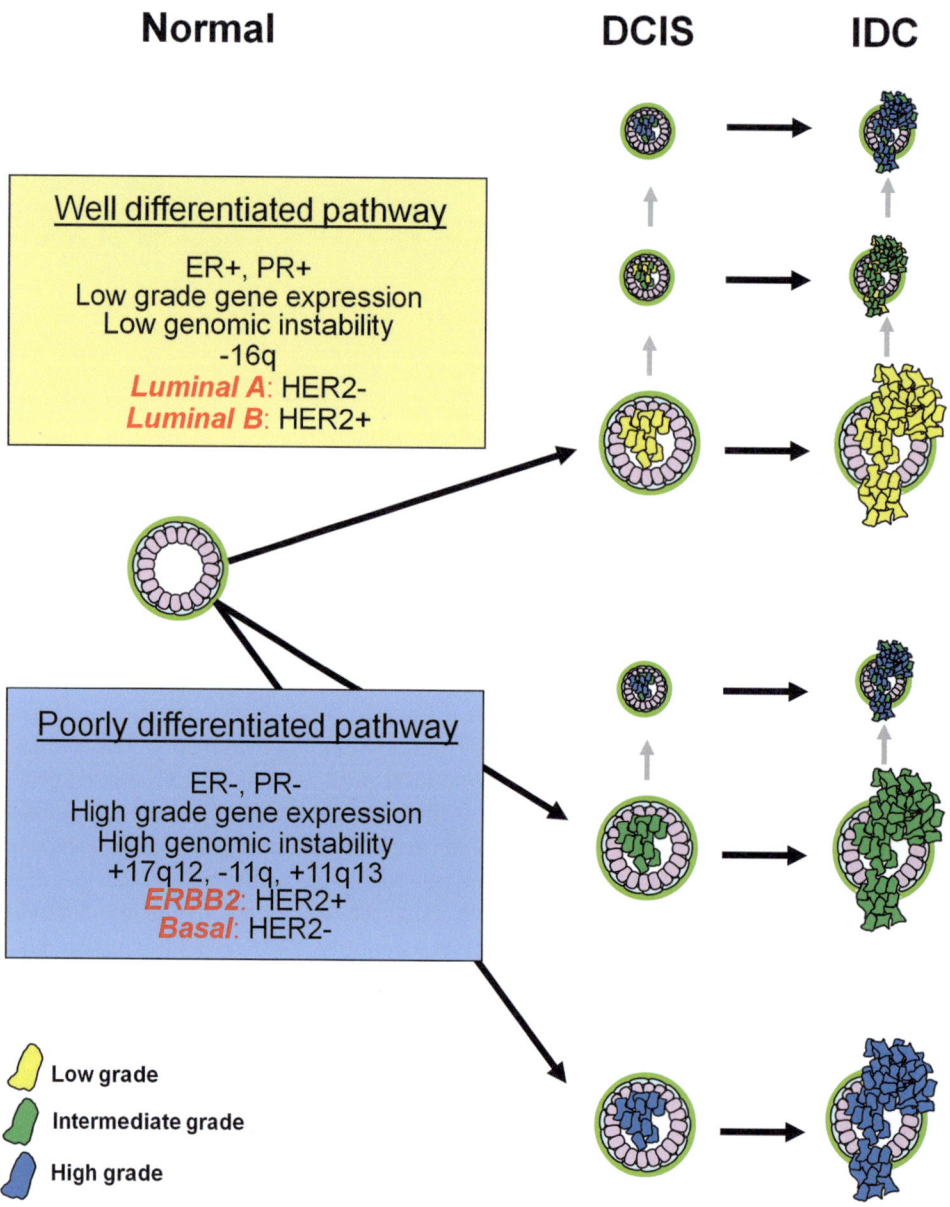

Normal **DCIS** **IDC**

Well differentiated pathway

ER+, PR+
Low grade gene expression
Low genomic instability
-16q
Luminal A: HER2-
Luminal B: HER2+

Poorly differentiated pathway

ER-, PR-
High grade gene expression
High genomic instability
+17q12, -11q, +11q13
ERBB2: HER2+
Basal: HER2-

Low grade
Intermediate grade
High grade

4   Future Directions and Challenges

The multi-pathway grade-specific model of DCIS progression appears to be qualitatively consistent with much, but not all, of the empirical data regarding DCIS. Recent studies have found prominent genomic changes during DCIS progression (Johnson et al. 2011; Knudsen et al. 2011; Hernandez et al. 2012), and evidence contrary to a low-grade pathway (King et al. 2011). To capture the complexity and heterogeneity of DCIS, it is likely that a combination of models will be necessary—sequential, precancer stem-cell, grade-specific, and others yet to be introduced. Additionally, it is critical for qualitative models of cancer progression to be augmented by mathematical approaches

to quantitatively test their predictive power. For example, Sontag et al. found that a parallel rather than linear mathematical model of DCIS progression to IDC was a better fit to co-occurrence data (Sontag and Axelrod 2005).

Clearly, there are many unanswered questions regarding the biology of DCIS and progression to invasive disease. These include the cell of origin responsible for preinvasive breast cancer, a more complete understanding of the DCIS to IDC transition including the complex interaction with the microenvironment, the proper placement of the intermediate grade phenotype in the evolution of DCIS, and the degree to which the fate of a preinvasive cancer is pre-encoded in its molecular/genetic/epigenetic phenotype. Addressing these outstanding questions is very challenging in patients because (i) the full natural history of DCIS cannot be

a Xenograft

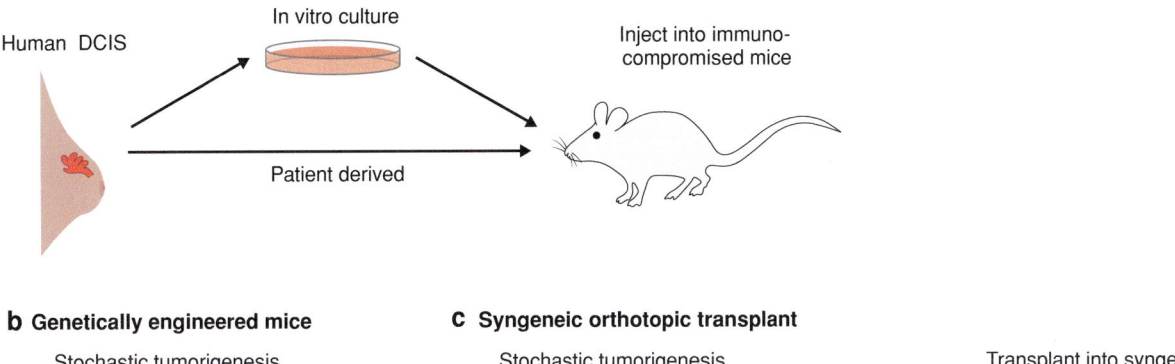

b Genetically engineered mice

Stochastic tumorigenesis

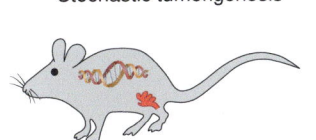

c Syngeneic orthotopic transplant

Stochastic tumorigenesis

Transplant into syngeneic mice

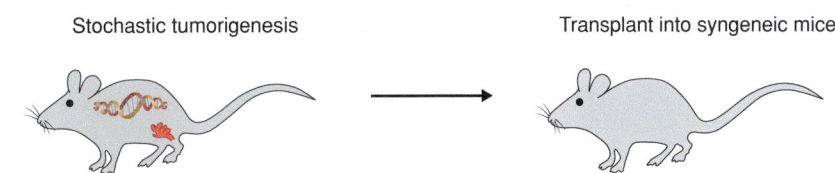

Fig. 6 Insights on DCIS progression from mouse models. **a** Xenograft models of DCIS use cells derived from human DCIS that are usually passaged in vitro many times before being injected into the mammary glands of immuno-compromised mice. MCF10DCIS and SUM-225 are the most commonly used established human DCIS cell lines and are injected either directly into the mammary fat pad or intraductally via the nipple (Miller et al. 2000; Behbod et al. 2009). Subsequently, DCIS develops and eventually progresses to invasive carcinoma. In work by Hu et al., co-injection of MCF10DCIS cells with myoepithelial cells suppressed DCIS progression, whereas co-injection with fibroblasts cells had a promoting effect, in part due to increased COX-2 expression (Hu et al. 2008, 2009). This highlights the importance of the microenvironment and suggests that loss of normal myoepithelial cell function is critical in promoting invasion. More recently, novel patient-derived xenograft models have been developed, wherein cells derived directly from freshly excised human DCIS are injected intraductally into immuno-compromised mice (Valdez et al. 2011), thereby recapitulating the diversity seen in human disease. **b** Genetically engineered mice (GEM) target genetic and molecular alterations implicated in human DCIS to arise specifically in the mammary glands of immuno-competent mice (Schulze-Garg et al. 2000; Maglione et al. 2001; Frech

et al. 2005; Li et al. 2008). High-grade mammary intraepithelial neoplasia (MIN) arising in these GEMs can resemble human DCIS (Cardiff et al. 2000) and precede the development of invasive carcinomas. An example is the C3(1) SV40 Tag model, wherein the Rb and p53 tumor suppressors are functionally inactivated (Maroulakou et al. 1994; Green et al. 2000). Serial MRI scans following MIN lesion development and progression over time in this model suggests that lesions have different latencies to progression, with some not progressing at all, even though they share the same genetic events (Jansen et al. 2009). This suggests that epigenetic or microenvironment factors influence invasive progression. **c** Syngeneic orthotopic transplant models collect tissue from MIN lesions in GEMs, serially transplant them in the cleared mammary fat pads of mice with the same genetic background and track progression to invasive cancer over time. Serial transplantation of individual MIN lesions arising in PyV-mT transgenic mice into FVB mice demonstrates that the distinct molecular characteristics and invasive potential of each MIN is stably maintained, and exhibits similar gene expression as its invasive stage (Maglione et al. 2001, 2004; Namba et al. 2004, 2006). This evidence supports the hypothesis that invasive potential and molecular characteristics are pre-encoded in DCIS (Damonte et al. 2008; Cardiff and Borowsky 2010)

tracked, due to obligate surgical excision, (ii) large cohorts are required, and (iii) long-term follow-up of patients must be linked to tissue repositories.

As an alternative to human studies, mouse model systems are an appealing experimental framework because in principle they do not suffer from the clinical limitations that confound human investigations. There are several types of DCIS models, including xenografts utilizing human DCIS cell lines injected into immuno-compromised mice (Miller et al. 2000; Behbod et al. 2009; Valdez et al. 2011), genetically engineered mice (GEM) that genetically disrupt pathways implicated in human DCIS (Green et al. 2000; Schulze-Garg et al. 2000; Maglione et al. 2001; Frech et al. 2005; Li et al. 2008), and orthotopic transplant models derived from GEM (Maglione et al. 2001, 2004; Medina et al. 2002; Namba et al. 2004, 2006; Damonte et al. 2008) (Fig. 6). Each type of

model has its advantages and disadvantages. Xenograft models are appealing because human cells or tissues are used, while GEM are excellent for modeling the stochastic events occurring during preinvasive cancer development and progression, within the context of an intact microenvironment. Such mouse models have already provided some important insights into DCIS (Fig. 6).

5 Summary

In examining the biology of DCIS, we have seen that important molecular pathways responsible for regulating cellular proliferation, apoptosis, and genome integrity are altered and exhibit marked inter- and intra-lesion heterogeneity. Yet the significance of these molecular signatures in terms of predicting risk of DCIS progression to invasive carcinoma is not fully known. We have found surprisingly few differences on a genomic or gene-expression level between DCIS and IDC. Yet the differences between grades and molecular subtypes of disease are profound, regardless of whether preinvasive or invasive, which led us to the multi-pathway grade-specific DCIS progression hypothesis. A question remains: how much of preinvasive breast cancer progression is predetermined, and how much is governed by stochastic events happening over time? Likely both are involved and very likely the microenvironment plays an important role. Improvements in molecular assays and model systems will provide further insights. From a clinical perspective, understanding the biology of DCIS and progression to invasive cancer is critical for achieving the important goal of identifying low-risk subsets of women that could benefit from less aggressive therapeutic interventions (Sorlie 2011). From a cancer biology perspective, focusing on this earliest stage of breast cancer can shed light on the origin breast cancer as well as the cancer pathways and mechanisms responsible for its progression.

Acknowledgments I would like to thank Dr. Amit Adhikari and the NIH Fellows Editorial Board for useful feedback.

References

Allegra CJ, Aberle DR, Ganschow P, Hahn SM, Lee CN, Millon-Underwood S, Pike MC, Reed SD, Saftlas AF, Scarvalone SA, Schwartz AM, Slomski C, Yothers G, Zon R (2010) National Institutes of Health state-of-the-science conference statement: diagnosis and management of ductal carcinoma in situ september 22–24, 2009. J Natl Cancer Inst 102:161–169

Allinen M, Beroukhim R, Cai L, Brennan C, Lahti-Domenici J, Huang H, Porter D, Hu M, Chin L, Richardson A, Schnitt S, Sellers WR, Polyak K (2004) Molecular characterization of the tumor microenvironment in breast cancer. Cancer Cell 6:17–32

Allred DC (2010) Ductal carcinoma in situ: terminology, classification, and natural history. J Natl Cancer Inst Monogr 2010:134–138

Allred DC, Wu Y, Mao S, Nagtegaal ID, Lee S, Perou CM, Mohsin SK, O'Connell P, Tsimelzon A, Medina D (2008) Ductal carcinoma in situ and the emergence of diversity during breast cancer evolution. Clin Cancer Res 14:370–378

Altintas S, Lambein K, Huizing MT, Braems G, Asjoe FT, Hellemans H, Van Marck E, Weyler J, Praet M, Van den Broecke R, Vermorken JB, Tjalma WA (2009) Prognostic significance of oncogenic markers in ductal carcinoma in situ of the breast: a clinicopathologic study. Breast J 15:120–132

Arun B, Vogel KJ, Lopez A, Hernandez M, Atchley D, Broglio KR, Amos CI, Meric-Bernstam F, Kuerer H, Hortobagyi GN, Albarracin CT (2009) High prevalence of preinvasive lesions adjacent to BRCA1/2-associated breast cancers. Cancer Prev Res (Phila) 2:122–127

Behbod F, Kittrell FS, LaMarca H, Edwards D, Kerbawy S, Heestand JC, Young E, Mukhopadhyay P, Yeh HW, Allred DC, Hu M, Polyak K, Rosen JM, Medina D (2009) An intraductal human-in-mouse transplantation model mimics the subtypes of ductal carcinoma in situ. Breast Cancer Res 11:R66

Bijker N, van Tienhoven G (2010) Local and systemic outcomes in DCIS based on tumor and patient characteristics: the radiation oncologist's perspective. J Natl Cancer Inst Monogr 2010:178–180

Boland GP, Butt IS, Prasad R, Knox WF, Bundred NJ (2004) COX-2 expression is associated with an aggressive phenotype in ductal carcinoma in situ. Br J Cancer 90:423–429

Bombonati A, Sgroi DC (2011) The molecular pathology of breast cancer progression. J Pathol 223:307–317

Bose S, Chandran S, Mirocha JM, Bose N (2006) The Akt pathway in human breast cancer: a tissue-array-based analysis. Mod Pathol 19:238–245

Buerger H, Otterbach F, Simon R, Poremba C, Diallo R, Decker T, Riethdorf L, Brinkschmidt C, Dockhorn-Dworniczak B, Boecker W (1999a) Comparative genomic hybridization of ductal carcinoma in situ of the breast-evidence of multiple genetic pathways. J Pathol 187:396–402

Buerger H, Otterbach F, Simon R, Schafer KL, Poremba C, Diallo R, Brinkschmidt C, Dockhorn-Dworniczak B, Boecker W (1999b) Different genetic pathways in the evolution of invasive breast cancer are associated with distinct morphological subtypes. J Pathol 189:521–526

Cardiff RD, Borowsky AD (2010) Precancer: sequentially acquired or predetermined? Toxicol Pathol 38:171–179

Cardiff RD, Anver MR, Gusterson BA, Hennighausen L, Jensen RA, Merino MJ, Rehm S, Russo J, Tavassoli FA, Wakefield LM, Ward JM, Green JE (2000) The mammary pathology of genetically engineered mice: the consensus report and recommendations from the Annapolis meeting. Oncogene 19:968–988

Chin K, de Solorzano CO, Knowles D, Jones A, Chou W, Rodriguez EG, Kuo WL, Ljung BM, Chew K, Myambo K, Miranda M, Krig S, Garbe J, Stampfer M, Yaswen P, Gray JW, Lockett SJ (2004) In situ analyses of genome instability in breast cancer. Nat Genet 36:984–988

Clark SE, Warwick J, Carpenter R, Bowen RL, Duffy SW, Jones JL (2011) Molecular subtyping of DCIS: heterogeneity of breast cancer reflected in pre-invasive disease. Br J Cancer 104:120–127

Claus EB, Petruzella S, Matloff E, Carter D (2005) Prevalence of BRCA1 and BRCA2 mutations in women diagnosed with ductal carcinoma in situ. JAMA 293:964–969

Correa C, McGale P, Taylor C, Wang Y, Clarke M, Davies C, Peto R, Bijker N, Solin L, Darby S (2010) Overview of the randomized trials of radiotherapy in ductal carcinoma in situ of the breast. J Natl Cancer Inst Monogr 2010:162–177

Damonte P, Hodgson JG, Chen JQ, Young LJ, Cardiff RD, Borowsky AD (2008) Mammary carcinoma behavior is programmed in the precancer stem cell. Breast Cancer Res: BCR 10:R50

D'Orsi CJ (2010) Imaging for the diagnosis and management of ductal carcinoma in situ. J Natl Cancer Inst Monogr 2010:214–217

Eng-Wong J, Costantino JP, Swain SM (2010) The impact of systemic therapy following ductal carcinoma in situ. J Natl Cancer Inst Monogr 2010:200–203

Erbas B, Provenzano E, Armes J, Gertig D (2006) The natural history of ductal carcinoma in situ of the breast: a review. Breast Cancer Res Treat 97:135–144

Espina V, Liotta LA (2011) What is the malignant nature of human ductal carcinoma in situ? Nat Rev Cancer 11:68–75

Frech MS, Halama ED, Tilli MT, Singh B, Gunther EJ, Chodosh LA, Flaws JA, Furth PA (2005) Deregulated estrogen receptor alpha expression in mammary epithelial cells of transgenic mice results in the development of ductal carcinoma in situ. Cancer Res 65:681–685

Gauthier ML, Berman HK, Miller C, Kozakeiwicz K, Chew K, Moore D, Rabban J, Chen YY, Kerlikowske K, Tlsty TD (2007) Abrogated response to cellular stress identifies DCIS associated with subsequent tumor events and defines basal-like breast tumors. Cancer Cell 12:479–491

Glover JA, Hughes CM, Cantwell MM, Murray LJ (2011) A systematic review to establish the frequency of cyclooxygenase-2 expression in normal breast epithelium, ductal carcinoma in situ, microinvasive carcinoma of the breast and invasive breast cancer. Br J Cancer 105:13–17

Green JE, Shibata MA, Yoshidome K, Liu ML, Jorcyk C, Anver MR, Wigginton J, Wiltrout R, Shibata E, Kaczmarczyk S, Wang W, Liu ZY, Calvo A, Couldrey C (2000) The C3(1)/SV40 T-antigen transgenic mouse model of mammary cancer: ductal epithelial cell targeting with multistage progression to carcinoma. Oncogene 19:1020–1027

Guidi AJ, Fischer L, Harris JR, Schnitt SJ (1994) Microvessel density and distribution in ductal carcinoma in situ of the breast. J Natl Cancer Inst 86:614–619

Hernandez L, Wilkerson PM, Lambros MB, Campion-Flora A, Rodrigues DN, Gauthier A, Cabral C, Pawar V, Mackay A, A'Hern R, Marchio C, Palacios J, Natrajan R, Weigelt B, Reis-Filho JS (2012) Genomic and mutational profiling of ductal carcinomas in situ and matched adjacent invasive breast cancers reveals intra-tumour genetic heterogeneity and clonal selection. J Pathol 227(1):42–52

Hieken TJ, Farolan M, D'Alessandro S, Velasco JM (2001) Predicting the biologic behavior of ductal carcinoma in situ: an analysis of molecular markers. Surgery 130:593–600 discussion 600–591

Hu M, Yao J, Cai L, Bachman KE, van den Brule F, Velculescu V, Polyak K (2005) Distinct epigenetic changes in the stromal cells of breast cancers. Nat Genet 37:899–905

Hu M, Yao J, Carroll DK, Weremowicz S, Chen H, Carrasco D, Richardson A, Violette S, Nikolskaya T, Nikolsky Y, Bauerlein EL, Hahn WC, Gelman RS, Allred C, Bissell MJ, Schnitt S, Polyak K (2008) Regulation of in situ to invasive breast carcinoma transition. Cancer Cell 13:394–406

Hu M, Peluffo G, Chen H, Gelman R, Schnitt S, Polyak K (2009) Role of COX-2 in epithelial-stromal cell interactions and progression of ductal carcinoma in situ of the breast. Proc Natl Acad Sci U S A 106:3372–3377

Hwang ES (2010) The impact of surgery on ductal carcinoma in situ outcomes: the use of mastectomy. J Natl Cancer Inst Monogr 2010:197–199

Hwang ES, DeVries S, Chew KL, Moore DH 2nd, Kerlikowske K, Thor A, Ljung BM, Waldman FM (2004) Patterns of chromosomal alterations in breast ductal carcinoma in situ. Clin Cancer Res 10:5160–5167

Hwang ES, McLennan JL, Moore DH, Crawford BB, Esserman LJ, Ziegler JL (2007) Ductal carcinoma in situ in BRCA mutation carriers. J Clin Oncol (Official Journal of the American Society of Clinical Oncology) 25:642–647

Jansen SA (2011) Ductal carcinoma in situ: detection, diagnosis, and characterization with magnetic resonance imaging. Semin Ultrasound CT MR 32:306–318

Jansen SA, Newstead GM, Abe H, Shimauchi A, Schmidt RA, Karczmar GS (2007) Pure ductal carcinoma in situ: kinetic and morphologic MR characteristics compared with mammographic appearance and nuclear grade. Radiology 245:684–691

Jansen SA, Conzen SD, Fan X, Markiewicz EJ, Newstead GM, Karczmar GS (2009) Magnetic resonance imaging of the natural history of in situ mammary neoplasia in transgenic mice: a pilot study. Breast Cancer Res 11:R65

Johnson CE, Gorringe KL, Thompson ER, Opeskin K, Boyle SE, Wang Y, Hill P, Mann GB, Campbell IG (2011) Identification of copy number alterations associated with the progression of DCIS to invasive ductal carcinoma. Breast Cancer Res Treat

Kane RL, Virnig BA, Shamliyan T, Wang SY, Tuttle TM, Wilt TJ (2010) The impact of surgery, radiation, and systemic treatment on outcomes in patients with ductal carcinoma in situ. J Natl Cancer Inst Monogr 2010:130–133

Kerlikowske K (2010) Epidemiology of ductal carcinoma in situ. J Natl Cancer Inst Monogr 2010:139–141

Kerlikowske K, Molinaro AM, Gauthier ML, Berman HK, Waldman F, Bennington J, Sanchez H, Jimenez C, Stewart K, Chew K, Ljung BM, Tlsty TD (2010) Biomarker expression and risk of subsequent tumors after initial ductal carcinoma in situ diagnosis. J Natl Cancer Inst 102:627–637

King TA, Sakr RA, Muhsen S, Andrade VP, Giri D, Van Zee KJ, Morrow M (2011) Is there a low-grade precursor pathway in breast cancer? Ann Surg Oncol 19:1115–1121

Knudsen ES, Ertel A, Davicioni E, Kline J, Schwartz GF, Witkiewicz AK (2011) Progression of ductal carcinoma in situ to invasive breast cancer is associated with gene expression programs of EMT and myoepithelia. Breast Cancer Res Treat

Kuerer HM, Albarracin CT, Yang WT, Cardiff RD, Brewster AM, Symmans WF, Hylton NM, Middleton LP, Krishnamurthy S, Perkins GH, Babiera G, Edgerton ME, Czerniecki BJ, Arun BK, Hortobagyi GN (2009) Ductal carcinoma in situ: state of the science and roadmap to advance the field. J Clin Oncol (Official Journal of the American Society of Clinical Oncology) 27:279–288

Kuhl CK, Schrading S, Bieling HB, Wardelmann E, Leutner CC, Koenig R, Kuhn W, Schild HH (2007) MRI for diagnosis of pure ductal carcinoma in situ: a prospective observational study. Lancet 370:485–492

Kulkarni S, Patil DB, Diaz LK, Wiley EL, Morrow M, Khan SA (2008) COX-2 and PPARgamma expression are potential markers of recurrence risk in mammary duct carcinoma in situ. BMC Cancer 8:36

Lari SA, Kuerer HM (2011) Biological markers in DCIS and risk of breast recurrence: a systematic review. J Cancer 2:232–261

Lehman CD (2010) Magnetic resonance imaging in the evaluation of ductal carcinoma in situ. J Natl Cancer Inst Monogr 2010:150–151

Li Y, Zhang Y, Hill J, Kim HT, Shen Q, Bissonnette RP, Lamph WW, Brown PH (2008) The rexinoid, bexarotene, prevents the development of premalignant lesions in MMTV-erbB2 mice. Br J Cancer 98:1380–1388

Livasy CA, Perou CM, Karaca G, Cowan DW, Maia D, Jackson S, Tse CK, Nyante S, Millikan RC (2007) Identification of a basal-like subtype of breast ductal carcinoma in situ. Human Pathol 38:197–204

Ma XJ, Salunga R, Tuggle JT, Gaudet J, Enright E, McQuary P, Payette T, Pistone M, Stecker K, Zhang BM, Zhou YX, Varnholt H, Smith B, Gadd M, Chatfield E, Kessler J, Baer TM, Erlander MG, Sgroi DC (2003) Gene expression profiles of human breast cancer progression. Proc Natl Acad Sci U S A 100:5974–5979

Ma XJ, Dahiya S, Richardson E, Erlander M, Sgroi DC (2009) Gene expression profiling of the tumor microenvironment during breast cancer progression. Breast Cancer Res: BCR 11:R7

Maglione JE, Moghanaki D, Young LJ, Manner CK, Ellies LG, Joseph SO, Nicholson B, Cardiff RD, MacLeod CL (2001) Transgenic polyoma middle-T mice model premalignant mammary disease. Cancer Res 61:8298–8305

Maglione JE, McGoldrick ET, Young LJ, Namba R, Gregg JP, Liu L, Moghanaki D, Ellies LG, Borowsky AD, Cardiff RD, MacLeod CL (2004) Polyomavirus middle T-induced mammary intraepithelial neoplasia outgrowths: single origin, divergent evolution, and multiple outcomes. Mol Cancer Ther 3:941–953

Maley CC, Galipeau PC, Finley JC, Wongsurawat VJ, Li X, Sanchez CA, Paulson TG, Blount PL, Risques RA, Rabinovitch PS, Reid BJ (2006) Genetic clonal diversity predicts progression to esophageal adenocarcinoma. Nat Genet 38:468–473

Maroulakou IG, Anver M, Garrett L, Green JE (1994) Prostate and mammary adenocarcinoma in transgenic mice carrying a rat C3(1) simian virus 40 large tumor antigen fusion gene. Proc Natl Acad Sci U S A 91:11236–11240

Marusyk A, Polyak K (2010) Tumor heterogeneity: causes and consequences. Biochim Biophys Acta 1805:105–117

Medina D, Kittrell FS, Shepard A, Stephens LC, Jiang C, Lu J, Allred DC, McCarthy M, Ullrich RL (2002) Biological and genetic properties of the p53 null preneoplastic mammary epithelium. FASEB J 16:881–883

Millar EK, Tran K, Marr P, Graham PH (2007) p27KIP-1, cyclin A and cyclin D1 protein expression in ductal carcinoma in situ of the breast: p27KIP-1 correlates with hormone receptor status but not with local recurrence. Pathol Int 57:183–189

Miller FR, Santner SJ, Tait L, Dawson PJ (2000) MCF10DCIS.com xenograft model of human comedo ductal carcinoma in situ. J Natl Cancer Inst 92:1185–1186

Namba R, Maglione JE, Young LJ, Borowsky AD, Cardiff RD, MacLeod CL, Gregg JP (2004) Molecular characterization of the transition to malignancy in a genetically engineered mouse-based model of ductal carcinoma in situ. Mol Cancer Res 2:453–463

Namba R, Maglione JE, Davis RR, Baron CA, Liu S, Carmack CE, Young LJ, Borowsky AD, Cardiff RD, Gregg JP (2006) Heterogeneity of mammary lesions represent molecular differences. BMC Cancer 6:275

Okumura Y, Yamamoto Y, Zhang Z, Toyama T, Kawasoe T, Ibusuki M, Honda Y, Iyama K, Yamashita H, Iwase H (2008) Identification of biomarkers in ductal carcinoma in situ of the breast with microinvasion. BMC Cancer 8:287

Perou CM, Sorlie T, Eisen MB, van de Rijn M, Jeffrey SS, Rees CA, Pollack JR, Ross DT, Johnsen H, Akslen LA, Fluge O, Pergamenschikov A, Williams C, Zhu SX, Lonning PE, Borresen-Dale AL, Brown PO, Botstein D (2000) Molecular portraits of human breast tumours. Nature 406:747–752

Polyak K (2007) Breast cancer: origins and evolution. J Clin Invest 117:3155–3163

Polyak K (2010) Molecular markers for the diagnosis and management of ductal carcinoma in situ. J Natl Cancer Inst Monogr 2010:210–213

Porter DA, Krop IE, Nasser S, Sgroi D, Kaelin CM, Marks JR, Riggins G, Polyak K (2001) A SAGE (serial analysis of gene expression) view of breast tumor progression. Cancer Res 61:5697–5702

Porter D, Lahti-Domenici J, Keshaviah A, Bae YK, Argani P, Marks J, Richardson A, Cooper A, Strausberg R, Riggins GJ, Schnitt S, Gabrielson E, Gelman R, Polyak K (2003) Molecular markers in ductal carcinoma in situ of the breast. Mol Cancer Res 1:362–375

Rakovitch E, Nofech-Mozes S, Hanna W, Narod S, Thiruchelvam D, Saskin R, Spayne J, Taylor C, Paszat L (2012) HER2/neu and Ki-67 expression predict non-invasive recurrence following breast-conserving therapy for ductal carcinoma in situ. Br J Cancer 106:1160–1165

Roylance R, Gorman P, Harris W, Liebmann R, Barnes D, Hanby A, Sheer D (1999) Comparative genomic hybridization of breast tumors stratified by histological grade reveals new insights into the biological progression of breast cancer. Cancer Res 59:1433–1436

Sardanelli F, Podo F, Santoro F, Manoukian S, Bergonzi S, Trecate G, Vergnaghi D, Federico M, Cortesi L, Corcione S, Morassut S, Di Maggio C, Cilotti A, Martincich L, Calabrese M, Zuiani C, Preda L, Bonanni B, Carbonaro LA, Contegiacomo A, Panizza P, Di Cesare E, Savarese A, Crecco M, Turchetti D, Tonutti M, Belli P, Maschio AD (2010) Multicenter surveillance of women at high genetic breast cancer risk using mammography, ultrasonography, and contrast-enhanced magnetic resonance imaging (the high breast cancer risk italian 1 study): final results. Invest Radiol 46:94–105

Schnitt SJ (2010) Local outcomes in ductal carcinoma in situ based on patient and tumor characteristics. J Natl Cancer Inst Monogr 2010:158–161

Schulze-Garg C, Lohler J, Gocht A, Deppert W (2000) A transgenic mouse model for the ductal carcinoma in situ (DCIS) of the mammary gland. Oncogene 19:1028–1037

Sgroi DC (2010) Preinvasive breast cancer. Ann Rev Pathol 5:193–221

Shamliyan T, Wang SY, Virnig BA, Tuttle TM, Kane RL (2010) Association between patient and tumor characteristics with clinical outcomes in women with ductal carcinoma in situ. J Natl Cancer Inst Monogr 2010:121–129

Smart CE, Simpson PT, Vargas AC, Lakhani SR (2011) Genetic alterations in normal and malignant breast tissue. In: Tot T (ed) Breast cancer: a lobar disease. Springer, London

Smith KL, Adank M, Kauff N, Lafaro K, Boyd J, Lee JB, Hudis C, Offit K, Robson M (2007) BRCA mutations in women with ductal carcinoma in situ. Clin Cancer Res (Official Journal of the American Association for Cancer Research) 13:4306–4310

Solin LJ (2010) The impact of adding radiation treatment after breast conservation surgery for ductal carcinoma in situ of the breast. J Natl Cancer Inst Monogr 2010:187–192

Sontag L, Axelrod DE (2005) Evaluation of pathways for progression of heterogeneous breast tumors. J Theor Biol 232:179–189

Sorlie T (2011) How to personalise treatment in early breast cancer. Eur J Cancer 47(Suppl 3):S310–S311

Sorlie T, Perou CM, Tibshirani R, Aas T, Geisler S, Johnsen H, Hastie T, Eisen MB, van de Rijn M, Jeffrey SS, Thorsen T, Quist H, Matese JC, Brown PO, Botstein D, Eystein Lonning P, Borresen-Dale AL (2001) Gene expression patterns of breast carcinomas distinguish tumor subclasses with clinical implications. Proc Natl Acad Sci U S A 98:10869–10874

Tamimi RM, Baer HJ, Marotti J, Galan M, Galaburda L, Fu Y, Deitz AC, Connolly JL, Schnitt SJ, Colditz GA, Collins LC (2008) Comparison of molecular phenotypes of ductal carcinoma in situ and invasive breast cancer. Breast Cancer Res 10:R67

Tot T (2010) The origins of early breast carcinoma. Semin Diagn Pathol 27:62–68

Tot T (2011) Subgross morphology, the sick lobe hypothesis, and the success of breast conservation. Int J Breast Cancer 2011:634021

Valdez KE, Fan F, Smith W, Allred DC, Medina D, Behbod F (2011) Human primary ductal carcinoma in situ (DCIS) subtype-specific pathology is preserved in a mouse intraductal (MIND) xenograft model. J Pathol 225:565–573

Vincent-Salomon A, Lucchesi C, Gruel N, Raynal V, Pierron G, Goudefroye R, Reyal F, Radvanyi F, Salmon R, Thiery JP, Sastre-Garau X, Sigal-Zafrani B, Fourquet A, Delattre O (2008) Integrated genomic and transcriptomic analysis of ductal carcinoma in situ of the breast. Clin Cancer Res 14:1956–1965

Virnig BA, Wang SY, Shamilyan T, Kane RL, Tuttle TM (2010) Ductal carcinoma in situ: risk factors and impact of screening. J Natl Cancer Inst Monogr 2010:113–116

Vogelstein B, Fearon ER, Hamilton SR, Kern SE, Preisinger AC, Leppert M, Nakamura Y, White R, Smits AM, Bos JL (1988) Genetic alterations during colorectal-tumor development. N Engl J Med 319:525–532

Warner E, Causer PA, Wong JW, Wright FC, Jong RA, Hill KA, Messner SJ, Yaffe MJ, Narod SA, Plewes DB (2011) Improvement in DCIS detection rates by MRI over time in a high-risk breast screening study. Breast J 17:9–17

Wellings SR, Jensen HM, Marcum RG (1975) An atlas of subgross pathology of the human breast with special reference to possible precancerous lesions. J Natl Cancer Inst 55:231–273

Witkiewicz AK, Rivadeneira DB, Ertel A, Kline J, Hyslop T, Schwartz GF, Fortina P, Knudsen ES (2011) Association of RB/p16-pathway perturbations with DCIS recurrence: dependence on tumor versus tissue microenvironment. Am J Pathol 179:1171–1178

Yu KD, Wu LM, Liu GY, Wu J, Di GH, Shen ZZ, Shao ZM (2011) Different distribution of breast cancer subtypes in breast ductal carcinoma in situ (DCIS), DCIS with microinvasion, and DCIS with invasion component. Ann Surg Oncol 18:1342–1348

Cancer Stem Cells and Radiotherapy

Jian Jian Li

Contents

Abstract

In clinic, tumor recurrence and metastasis are the major barriers to further improve the overall cancer patients' survival. The theory of tumor repopulation due to radiation described decades ago is being supported by new experimental data. The heterogeneity of cancer cell populations in a given tumor is recently evidenced by the present of cancer stem cells (CSCs) that are different from other non-CSC tumor cells and maintain unique self-renewal and tumor-initiating phenotypes. The CSCs isolated from many human tumors including the breast cancer stem cells (BCSCs) are demonstrated to hold specific characteristics and are demonstrated to be resistant to an array of anti-cancer agents and radiation therapy. In this chapter, a number of prosurvival pathways and biomarkers found in BCSCs will be discussed. Several prosurvival features including CSCs repopulation, DNA repair ability, as well as the HER2-NFκB-HER2 signaling loop in the radioresistant BCSCs will be illustrated. Further clarification of the specific networks associated with the radioresistant phenotype of BCSCs will shed new light on the molecular mechanism of tumor radioresistance, and will help to generate targets to detect and treat therapy-resistant tumor cells.

1 Introduction

Despite a trend toward overall improvement in early detection and therapy outcomes, breast cancer (BC) mortality remains unacceptably high, especially for patients with recurrent or metastatic tumors (Lacroix 2006). Recent data suggest that tumors contain cancer stem cells (CSCs) which play an integral role in tumor growth and resistance to treatment. The CSC classification emerges from data showing that only a small proportion of tumor cells are able to form colonies or new tumors (Bonnet and Dick 1997; Al-Hajj et al. 2003). Specific cell surface markers such as

J. J. Li (✉)
Department of Radiation Oncology,
University of California Davis, 4501 X Street,
Sacramento, CA 95817, USA
e-mail: jian-jian.li@ucdmc.ucdavis.edu

J. Strauss et al. (eds.), *Breast Cancer Biology for the Radiation Oncologist*, Medical Radiology. Radiation Oncology,
DOI: 10.1007/174_2012_648, © Springer-Verlag Berlin Heidelberg 2012
Published Online: 19 June 2012

CD44$^+$/CD24$^{-/low}$ in breast cancer stem cells (BCSCs) (Al-Hajj et al. 2003) are shown to have increased expression of pro-invasive genes required for metastasis such as IL-1α, IL-6, IL-8, and urokinase plasminogen activator (Sheridan et al. 2006). Additionally, CSCs appear to exhibit notable radioresistance. In tumor cells under genotoxic stress conditions (such as ionizing radiation), activation of pro-survival pathways and inhibition of pro-apoptotic pathways are responsible for tumor radioresistance. The molecules involved in these pathways are potential targets to enhance tumor radiosensitivity. Clinical data suggest that breast cancer patients with tumors overexpressing HER2/neu, a member of ErbB family of receptor tyrosine kinases, show a poor prognosis compared to HER2/neu negative tumors, and the HER2 gene enhancement is correlated with the time to relapse of the disease (Slamon et al. 1987). The poorer prognosis of women with Her2/Neu amplified tumors is entirely abrogated if they are treated with anti-HER2 therapy. Upon irradiation, cells overexpressing HER2 are able to activate NFκB, a key transcription factor in stress response that regulates a pro-survival network (Guo et al. 2004). Importantly, the NFκB binding motif in the HER2 gene promoter region is found to be responsible for radiation-induced HER2 expression (Cao et al. 2009). Defining the central role of NFκB in these pathways may offer new therapeutic targets for breast cancer treatment. This chapter will focus on CSCs, tumor radioresistance, and the role of NFκB-Her2 in mediating radioresistance, with an emphasis on experimental laboratory data. Clarification of such prosurvival networks activated in CSCs will not only help to develop effective targets to sensitize tumor cells to radiotherapy, but also generate specific diagnostic approaches for the detection of recurrent or metastatic tumors.

2 CSC-Mediated Tumor Repopulation

Tumor resistance to radiotherapy and chemotherapy poses serious challenges to current cancer treatments including breast cancer therapies (Stockler et al. 2000). Increased tumorigenicity of CSCs with specific surface markers was first studied in acute myeloid leukemia (Bonnet and Dick 1997; Pardal et al. 2003). A CSC is thus defined as a specific tumor cell that has stem-cell like properties including the capacity to self-renew and to generate the heterogeneous lineages of cancer cells that comprise the tumor. A key feature of CSC theory is that only a small subset of tumor cells has the ability to proliferate in an uncontrolled manner (Al-Hajj et al. 2003; Al-Hajj 2007; Dalerba et al. 2007; Hurt et al. 2008). CSC theory challenges the transitional assumption that each tumor cell is capable of renewing the entire tumor. Al-Hajj et al. demonstrated that breast cancer cells expressing CD44 (CD44$^+$) but not CD24 (CD24$^{-/low}$)

are more tumorigenic; as few as 100 cells with this phenotype are able to form tumors in mice, while millions of cells without this feature cannot. These results suggest that CD44$^+$/CD24$^{-/low}$ may be a marker of breast CSCs (Al-Hajj et al. 2003). However, expression of the CD44$^+$/CD24$^{-/low}$ feature alone is not sufficient for the spread of breast cancer (Sheridan et al. 2006), suggesting there is great complexity of CSCs and their biomarkers. Recent work has demonstrated that the inhibition of aldehyde dehydrogenase (ALDH) activity reduces chemotherapy and radiation resistance of stem-like ALDH(hi)CD44 (+) human breast cancer cells (Croker and Allan 2011), indicating that ALDH and other prosurvival molecules may be required for the aggressive growth of BCSCs (Ginestier et al. 2007). Although many aspects of CSCs remain to be elucidated, accumulating evidence suggests that CSCs are present in many kinds of human cancer and may be associated with tumor reoccurrence, aggressiveness, and therapy-resistance.

Long-term observations of irradiated cells using computerized video time-lapse analyses reveal alternative cell fates other than apoptosis. The outcomes among irradiated tumor cells vary by the timing of induction and execution of cell death in cells with the same genomic background (Prieur-Carrillo et al. 2003; Forrester et al. 2000). This is strong evidence indicating that a tumor population previously thought to be homogeneous, in fact, contains different subpopulations with divergent behaviors. As an example, breast cancer MCF7 cells appear to be part of a heterogeneous population and the individual clones—derived after irradiation with fractionated doses—show varied radiosensitivities (Li et al. 2001). These observations are compatible with the idea that CSCs are more radioresistant than the non-stem cells (Baumann et al. 2008).

Repopulation of cancer cells during, or after completion of, anticancer therapy has long been considered the cause of treatment failure (Kim and Tannock 2005). Bao et al. (2006) report that glioma stem cells are able to promote radioresistance by enhancing DNA damage repair. Phillips et al. grew CD44$^+$/CD24$^{-/low}$ cancer-initiating cells isolated from breast cancer cell lines MCF7 and MDA-MB-231; these cells were found to propagate as mammospheres, a behavior that may explain their relative radioresistance (Phillips et al. 2006). Using the model of xenogeneic tumors treated with chemotherapy, Dylla et al. identified the repopulation of colorectal CSCs with the marker of CD44+ ESA+ (Dylla et al. 2008). These authors demonstrated that after anticancer therapy, the remaining colon cancer cell population is enriched for CSCs and thus, the remaining cells are more tumorigenic (Dylla et al. 2008). Importantly, enrichment of a tumor cell population for CSCs has been supported clinically. In clinical study, the proportion of putative CSCs in a residual tumor has been shown to increase following cytotoxic chemotherapy

(Diehn et al. 2009). The resistance of stem cells to cytoxic therapy, at least in some cell lines, may relate to the presence of a subset of quiescent CSCs that are more treatment-resistant than rapidly dividing cells (Diehn et al. 2009). The existence of different subclones of CSCs with varied sets of mutations and genomic alterations may be likely since heterogenous tumors consist of unstable genomes. During chemo- and/or radio- therapy, the most resistant CSCs would be selected and continue to sustain the tumor. These findings shed light onto a new conceptual paradigm of how CSCs or tumor-initiating cells contribute to the radiation response. Identification of CSC-associated radioresistance needs to be further evaluated in clinical studies.

3 Enhanced DNA Repair in CSC Radioresistance

It has long been proposed that a balance between the degree of DNA damage and activation of pro-survival signaling pathways determines the fate of an irradiated cell (Wolff 1989; Weichselbaum et al. 1994; Maity et al. 1997; Waldman et al. 1997; Schmidt-Ullrich et al. 2000). Some irradiated cells are also able to increase their survival rate by reducing or repairing radiation-induced damage via the activation of stress responsive signaling networks controlled by several radiation-inducible transcription factors including NFκB (Stecca and Gerber 1998; Wolff 1998; Feinendegen 1999; Li et al. 2001; Feinendegen 2002; Guo et al. 2003). The induced protection/tolerance of irradiated cells is especially evident when a cell is pre-exposed to a low or intermediate dose of x- or γ-rays, which can reduce the lethal effects and genomic instability caused by subsequent exposure to higher doses of radiation (Wolff 1989; Olivieri et al. 1984; Kelsey et al. 1991; Suzuki et al. 1998; Skov 1999; Robson et al. 2000; Suzuki et al. 2001). In this case, the activation of a survival network by an initial exposure to radiation is protective against the potentially lethal effects of a subsequent exposure.

The activation of the survival responses leading to a lower rate of apoptosis in CSCs is thought to be one of the major mechanisms for the resistance of cancer stem cells to radiation and chemotherapy (Frosina 2009). The increased capacity of CSCs for DNA repair (Johannessen et al. 2008) accounts for their low rate of apoptosis in response to cancer treatment. Glioma stem cells are able to promote radioresistance by enhancing DNA damage repair and reducing the rate of apoptosis following the repopulation of CD133$^+$ tumor cells after irradiation (Bao et al. 2006). Furthermore, CD133$^+$ glioma cells are shown to survive radiation by preferentially activating DNA damage checkpoints, repairing the radiation-induced DNA damage more effectively, and thus undergoing apoptosis less frequently than CD133$^-$ cells. After radiation treatment, increased activation of DNA damage checkpoint proteins is observed in CD133$^+$ cells, which ensures more efficient DNA repair in these cells. The addition of inhibitors specific for Chk1 and Chk2 checkpoint kinases are shown to radiosensitize the radioresistant CD133$^+$ glioma cells (Bao et al. 2006). It may be that the transient activation of the DNA checkpoints leads to cell cycle arrest, a required step for the initiation of DNA repair process. An interesting conclusion derived from these studies is that increased activation of checkpoint proteins, with no associated change in protein expression, is detected in cancer stem cells in response to radiation-induced DNA damage. This suggests the involvement of other mechanisms to regulate checkpoint activity and the survival of the cancer stem cells (Rich 2007).

Accumulating evidence reveals the relationship between radioresistance and DNA repair and cell cycle control via a variety of mechanisms that involve several signaling pathways (Puc et al. 2005; Skvortsova 2008). It is important to clarify if these mechanisms are activated more in the CSCs. Skvortsova et al. suggests that glyceraldehyde-3-phosphate dehydrogenase (GAPDH) and phosphoglycerate kinase 1 (PGK1) have roles in both DNA replication and repair in mammalian cells (Skvortsova 2008). Moreover, PGK1 is identified as a downstream effector in HER2 signaling and contributes to the aggressiveness of the breast cancer. Additionally, DNA-(apurinic or apyrimidinic site) lyase (APEX1) is also found to be upregulated in radioresistant prostate cancer cells and it is shown to have a role in DNA damage repair via the regulation of several transcription factors including NFκB (Skvortsova 2008). In addition, PTEN function is important for the localization of Chk1 and the loss of PTEN leads to genetic instability (Puc et al. 2005), contributing to the radioresistance of glioma cells (Jiang et al. 2007). Interestingly, loss of PTEN has also been associated with the induction of NFκB, a transcriptional suppressor of PTEN, via PI3 K/Akt pathway, which is suggested to be involved in chemoresistance in acute lymphoblastic leukemia cell lines (Guo et al. 2004). In addition to PI3 K/Akt pathway, NFκB can be activated by other signaling pathways including Ras/MAPK induced by several cytokines, growth factors and tyrosine kinases. NFκB activation is a transient process that has to be tightly regulated in order to avoid over-enhancing cell survival. In tumor cells, deregulation of different signaling pathways as well as alterations in the activity or the expression of several genes may lead to the disregulation of NFκB, enabling its constitutive activity. There are genes involved in cell cycle control, migration, adhesion, and apoptosis among the NFκB target genes (Dolcet et al. 2005). Lavon et al. reported the original observation indicating a role of NFκB in the regulation of DNA repair mechanisms. O^6-Methyl-guanine-DNA-Methyltransferase (MGMT) is a DNA repair enzyme responsible for resistance to several alkylating agents, thus conferring chemoresistance to certain tumor types (Lavon et al. 2007; Margison et al. 2003). Elevated activity of MGTM has been detected in many types of tumors including breast cancer, although the levels of activation are variable and even absent in some tumors (Margison et al. 2003). In glioma cell lines, the activity of NFκB is associated with the expression of MGTM (Lavon et al. 2007). Further experiments showed that NFκB is a major player in the regulation of MGTM, suggesting a new model for the mechanism of DNA damage repair mediated by NFκB upon exposure to alkylating agents (Lavon et al. 2007). Based on these data, it is plausible to posit that there is an orchestrated response of activation of NFκB regulated DNA damage checkpoint proteins in radioresistant CSCs. Further studies are needed to determine if this relation is exclusive to CSCs and whether it contributes significantly to clinical radioresistance.

4   Other Prosurvival Signaling Network in CSCs

Therapeutic radiation not only causes DNA damage but also generates oxidative stress, both of which can activate specific signaling pathways in an irradiated cell (Spitz et al. 2004). Depending on the extent of DNA damage, either pro-apoptotic or pro-survival pathways can be initiated. Studies of glioma CSCs give a general idea about the complex regulation of CSCs. Several pathways including the activation of receptor tyrosine kinases (RTKs), Bone Morphogenetic Proteins (BMPRs), Hedgehog and Notch are shown to be important for governing glioma CSCs. EGFR, a member of RTK family, is shown to play a significant role in proliferation and neurosphere formation in glioma CSCs. Activation of pro-survival AKT/phosphoinositide 3-hydroxykinase pathway, which is downstream of RTKs, has been shown to be more dominant in glioma CSCs compared to non-stem glioma cells. Hedgehog pathway is reported to be active in gliomas, and it has been suggested that it is necessary for self-renewal of CSCs (Li et al. 2009). It has been proposed that after irradiation at least three different populations of tumor cells exhibit differing responses. The main tumor cell population, which is radiosensitive, undergoes p53-dependent apoptosis, whereas the other two cell populations are radioresistant. The CSC population will undergo p53-dependent cell cycle arrest allowing for DNA repair. The non-proliferating tumor cell population does not respond to radiation at all (Hambardzumyan et al. 2008). Phillips et al. (2006) showed that NOTCH signaling pathway is activated in breast CSCs through PI3 K pathway upon exposure to radiation. Their study indicates that the CSC population is enriched in breast cancer via NOTCH

signaling pathway which is activated by radiation (Phillips et al. 2006). Several genes, including HER2, which is related to radioresistance, cyclinD1, CDK2, and NOTCH-4 have been identified to be upregulated via activation of NOTCH-1 signaling (Phillips et al. 2006). Downregulation of SirT1 (silencing information regulator) has been shown to enhance the radiosensitivity in prostate cancer cell and in CD133$^+$ glioblastoma cells, which are believed to be the brain cancer stem cells. SirT1 can physically bind to many proteins and interact with several pathways including p53, NFκB, and ATM (Chang et al. 2009). Thus, it is clear that many complex signaling pathways are involved in the maintenance, tumorigenicity and radio-resistance of CSCs.

5   NFκB-Initiated Pro-survival Network

NFκB is a sequence-specific gene regulator involved in inflammation and carcinogenesis and one of the major transcription factors activated by DNA damage stress in mammalian cells (Baldwin 1996; Karin 2006). The major NFκB components, p65 and p50, form a heterodimer that remains inactive in the cytoplasm in association with its inhibitor, IκB. The phosphorylation, dissociation, and proteolysis of IκB are mediated by the IKK (the IκB kinase) complex that contains two catalytic subunits, IKKα/IKK1 and IKKβ/IKK2, and a regulatory subunit IKKγ/NEMO (NFκB essential modulator). Upon release by IκB, NFκB is free to translocate to the nucleus and regulate the expression of its target genes (Lenardo and Baltimore 1989; Granville et al. 2000; Li and Verma 2002). Apart from its role in carcinogenesis, NFκB is shown to prevent apoptosis in transformed cells and enhance survival in many types of cancers (Jung et al. 1995; Baldwin 2001; Tang et al. 2001; Kataoka et al. 2002; Gilmore 2003; Kucharczak et al. 2003; Danial and Korsmeyer 2004). Not surprisingly, NFκB controlled effector genes play a role in cellular response to low or high doses of radiation (Brach et al. 1991; Luo et al. 2005; Fan et al. 2007). Radiation-induced NFκB activation can be mediated via the nuclear DNA damage through activation of DNA damage sensor protein ATM (Ataxia Telangiectasia Mutated). The ATM protein in turn activates the SUMO (small ubiquitin-like modifier) pathway that sumoylates another factor, NEMO, resulting in its nuclear translocation and subsequent association with ATM in the nucleus. ATM-dependent phosphorylation causes the nuclear export of NEMO and activation of the typical pathway (Curry et al. 1999; Locke et al. 2002). This is a very important finding that established the mechanism of activation of cytoplasmic stress sensors like NFκB by DNA damage signals that are predominant in the nucleus of an irradiated cell.

Many studies have investigated the effects of the inhibition of NFκB activity in the radiation response. Inhibition of NFκB has been shown to modulate ATM-associated apoptosis (Jung and Dritschilo 2001; Jung et al. 1997) and notably to enhance heat-mediated radiosensitization (Curry et al. 1999; Locke et al. 2002). However, blocking NFκB activity results in different effects in a tumor that is receiving radiation treatment. This may be related to many different NFkB effector genes involved in a wide array of physiological functions (Barkett and Gilmore 1999; Romashkova and Makarov 1999). Therefore, more specific NFκB effector genes that mediate the survival response after irradiation, especially those in tumor-acquired radioresistance and/or radiation-resistant cancer stem cells, need to be identified in order to understand the specificity of the response and linked pathophysiology. Importantly, the NFκB signaling network might be activated in breast cancer stem cells (Diehn et al. 2009). NFκB can be activated via HER2 overexpression and subsequently cause more overexpression of HER2 in breast cancer cells that have the radioresistant phenotype (Cao et al. 2009). We believe that these findings are exciting because they may indicate the existence of a very elegant survival strategy used specifically by cancer stem cells. Future studies should include experiments with live sorting of cancer cells in order to obtain CSCs and be used to confirm that this loop is actually activated only in the cancer stem cells upon radiation exposure.

6   HER2 and Breast Cancer Radioresistance

The HER2 proto-oncogene, which is located in the long arm of human chromosome 17 and encodes a 185 kD transmembrane glycoprotein in various tissues of epithelial, mesenchymal, and neuronal origin (Soomro et al. 1991; Olayioye 2001), belongs to the ErbB family of receptor tyrosine kinases. The ErbB family of receptor tyrosine kinases is composed of four members; the Epidermal Growth Factor receptor (EGFR) ErB1/HER1, ErbB2/HER2/Neu, ErbB3/HER3, and ErbB4/HER4 (Citri and Yarden 2006). Signal transduction is initiated by an agonist binding to the extracellular domain of an ErbB receptor followed by receptor dimerization and trans-autophosphorylation of specific tyrosine residues within the cytoplasmic domain. The phosphorylated receptor recruits downstream signaling proteins that contain Src homology 2 (SH2) and phosphotyrosine binding (PTB) domains that have a high affinity for phosphotyrosine residues. There is no known soluble ligand for HER2 but it is still very important because of its strong kinase activity and the fact that it is the preferred dimerization partner of other ErbB family members (Citri and Yarden 2006; Warren and Landgraf 2006). Moreover, HER2 can spontaneously form homodimers and automatically phosphorylate itself to obtain intrinsic tyrosine kinase

activity (Eccles 2001). The binding of specific effector proteins to the activated receptor leads to the activation of many different signaling pathways including Ras–mitogen-activated protein kinase (Ras-MAPK), phosphatidylinositol 3'kinase-protein kinase B (PI3 K-PKB/Akt) and phospholipase C–protein kinase C (PLC-PKC) pathways and enables receptor coupling to biological responses (Warren and Landgraf 2006). Not surprisingly, altered ErbB signaling has been shown to be involved in cancer development and progression as it is responsible for regulating proliferation, survival and/or differentiation by activating multiple signal transduction pathways (Warren and Landgraf 2006; Britten 2004).

Depending on the type of breast cancer, up to one-third of breast cancers show HER2 overexpression or gene amplification and individual tumor cells can have more than 2 million HER2 receptors (Haffty et al. 1996; Valabrega et al. 2007). HER2 overexpression is associated with aggressive tumor growth, resistance to treatment, metastasis and a high risk of local relapse and recurrence resulting in poor prognosis (Slamon et al. 1987; Haffty et al. 1996; Holbro et al. 2003). HER2 is linked to BCSCs (Diehn et al. 2009) and is valuable both as a prognostic marker and as a predictive factor for response to targeted agents to the Her-2 pathway (Haffty et al. 1996; Hicks et al. 2005). Research on ErbB family members and their involvement in cancer development and progression led scientists to develop antibodies against some individual members. The anti-HER2 monoclonal antibody, rhumAbHER2 (trastuzamab/herceptin) is the first of anticancer agents suppressing HER2 expression (Uno et al. 2001). It is the humanized form of the murine 4D5 antibody that is directed to the external domain of HER2, inhibiting growth of the cells with HER2 overexpression and was approved by FDA as both an adjuvant therapy in conjunction with chemotherapy and to be used in the setting of metastatic breast cancer overexpressing HER2 (Slamon et al. 2001; Liang et al. 2003). Herceptin, which has been shown to inhibit proliferation of breast cancer cells, also promotes the radiation-induced apoptosis and, depending on the level of HER2 overexpression, radiosensitizes cancer cells (Liang et al. 2003).

HER2 overexpression induces mammary carcinogenesis, tumor growth and invasion affecting normal and malignant mammary stem cells (Korkaya et al. 2008). It has been found that stem/progenitor cells increase in normal mammary epithelial cells upon overexpression of HER2. Moreover, the tumorigenicity of mammary cell lines is enhanced when HER2 is present and this group of cells shows an increased frequency of aldehyde dehydrogenase 1 (ALDH1)-positive cells (Diehn et al. 2009). These data are significant given that ALDH1 is suggested as a CSC marker, including breast cancer (Ginestier et al. 2007; Diehn et al. 2009).

Fig. 1 a The ROS and nuclear DNA damages induced by radiation can activate NFκB that in turn enters into the nucleus and binds to the promoter of HER2 gene causing its transactivation. The increased HER2 protein copies further activate NFκB activity thus accelerating the HER2-NFκB-HER2 loop, which is simplified and shown in b

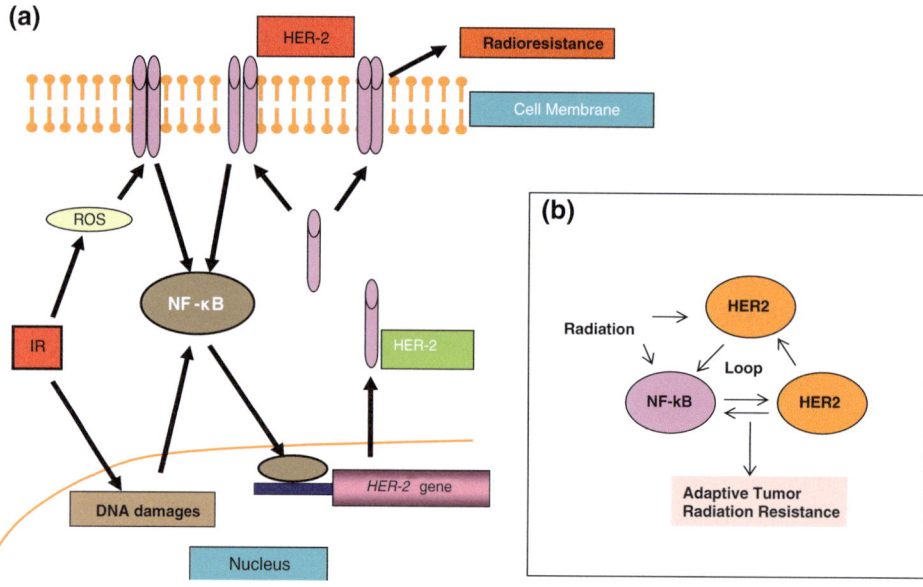

7   NFκB and HER2 Crosstalk in Signaling Breast Cancer Radioresistance

HER2 overexpression influences the response to radiotherapy but the key elements mediating HER2-radioresistance have not been well established (Summers et al. 1989). Overexpression of HER2 not only increases cell proliferation and survival (Kurokawa and Arteaga 2001), but also causes NFκB activation via PI3 K/Akt pathway, which can be inhibited by the tumor suppressor phosphatase PTEN (Pianetti et al. 2001). NFκB and its regulated genes are activated in breast cancer MCF7 cells with HER2 overexpression (Guo et al. 2004). MCF7 cells overexpressing HER2 are resistant to radiation-induced apoptosis with increased post-radiation clonogenic survival (Liang et al. 2003; Pietras et al. 1999). Overexpression of HER2 enhances NFκB activation while stable transfection of mutant IκB (MCF7/HER2/mIκB) or treatment with Herceptin inhibits NFκB activity and radiosensitizes MCF7 cells (Guo et al. 2004). Moreover, it has been found that Akt is required for HER2-mediated NFκB activation in radiation response (Guo et al. 2004). Liang et al. suggests that the MAPK and PI3 K/Akt pathways are involved in HER2-mediated resistance to radiation-induced apoptosis in breast cancer cells (Liang et al. 2003). Akt-mediated NFκB activation blocks apoptosis in HER2-expressing cells (Yang et al. 2000). Taken together, it is highly possible that NFκB and HER2 are mutually dependent in the activation of a prosurvival signaling pathway in irradiated breast cancer and other human cancer cells. Importantly, the HER2-negative cancer cells such as MCF7 cells that do not express HER2, may be induced to express HER2 and thus related to

tumor adaptive radioresistance (Guo et al. 2004; Cao et al. 2009). Accumulating data also demonstrate that radiation-induced NFκB regulates HER2 overexpression in radioresistant breast cancer cells selected from FIR-derived heterogenic population. These results demonstrate a loop-like pathway of HER2-NFκB-HER2 induced in tumor adaptive radioresistance (Fig. 1a, b). It would be important to answer the question of whether the HER2-NFκB-HER2 loop is specifically conjugated with CD44$^+$/CD24$^{-/low}$ and other biomarkers of BCSCs. Identification of this loop in BCSC radioresistance may generate new therapeutic targets to sensitize BCSCs and other cancer stem cells to radiotherapy.

8   Conclusion

Accumulating experimental evidence supports the existence of a subpopulation of cancer cells known as cancer stem cells (CSCs). These cells comprise a small portion of most tumors and are uniquely able to regenerate an entire tumor. This population of cells may express different cell surface markers than most other tumor cells; in breast cancer, some evidence suggests that CSCs exhibit a CD44$^+$/CD24$^{-/}$phenotype. In addition to their role as a progenitor population, CSCs appear to be especially resistant to anticancer therapies, including radiotherapy. The radio-resistance of CSCs appears to be mediated by both the activation of pro-survival pathways and the inhibition of pro-apoptotic pathways. Early data suggest that activation of the NFκB pathway is integral to radio-resistance: NFκB initiates a pro-survival pathway by enhancing DNA repair through the control of cell cycle checkpoints, and NFκB also contributes to radio-resistance through the inhibition of apoptosis. Importantly, the NFκB pathway is initiated by the HER2 signaling pathway, itself an important therapeutic target in breast cancer. There is emerging evidence that NFκB may feedback to enhance HER2 signaling, a positive feedback mechanism dubbed the HER2-NFκB-HER2 loop. The molecular mechanisms underlying CSC-related radio-resistance are not yet fully elucidated. It is hoped that clarification of these pathways will yield insights into the design of pharmaceuticals to overcome radio-resistance (and chemo-resistance) and render the all-important CSCs vulnerable to cytotoxic therapies.

References

Al-Hajj M (2007) Cancer stem cells and oncology therapeutics. Curr Opin Oncol 19:61–64

Al-Hajj M, Wicha MS, Benito-Hernandez A, Morrison SJ, Clarke MF (2003) Prospective identification of tumorigenic breast cancer cells. Proc Natl Acad Sci U S A 100:3983–3988

Baldwin AS (1996) The NFkappa B and I kappa B proteins: new discoveries and insights. Annu Rev Immunol 14:649–683

Baldwin AS (2001) Control of oncogenesis and cancer therapy resistance by the transcription factor NFkappaB. J Clin Invest 107:241–246

Bao S, Wu Q, McLendon RE, Hao Y, Shi Q, Hjelmeland AB, Dewhirst MW, Bigner DD, Rich JN (2006) Glioma stem cells promote radioresistance by preferential activation of the DNA damage response. Nature 444:756–760

Barkett M, Gilmore TD (1999) Control of apoptosis by Rel/NFkappaB transcription factors. Oncogene 18:6910–6924

Baumann M, Krause M, Hill R (2008) Exploring the role of cancer stem cells in radioresistance. Nat Rev Cancer 8:545–554

Bonnet D, Dick JE (1997) Human acute myeloid leukemia is organized as a hierarchy that originates from a primitive hematopoietic cell. Nat Med 3:730–737

Brach MA, Hass R, Sherman ML, Gunji H, Weichselbaum R, Kufe D (1991) Ionizing radiation induces expression and binding activity of the nuclear factor kappa B. J Clin Invest 88:691–695

Britten CD (2004) Targeting ErbB receptor signaling: a pan-ErbB approach to cancer. Mol Cancer Ther 3:1335–1342

Cao N, Li S, Wang Z, Ahmed KM, Degnan ME, Fan M, Dynlacht JR, Li JJ (2009) NFkappaB-mediated HER2 overexpression in radiation-adaptive resistance. Radiat Res 171:9–21

Chang CJ, Hsu CC, Yung MC, Chen KY, Tzao C, Wu WF, Chou HY, Lee YY, Lu KH, Chiou SH, Ma HI (2009) Enhanced radiosensitivity and radiation-induced apoptosis in glioma CD133-positive cells by knockdown of SirT1 expression. Biochem Biophys Res Commun 380:236–242

Citri A, Yarden Y (2006) EGF-ERBB signalling: towards the systems level. Nat Rev Mol Cell Biol 7:505–516

Croker AK, Allan AL (2011). Inhibition of aldehyde dehydrogenase (ALDH) activity reduces chemotherapy and radiation resistance of stem-like ALDH(hi)CD44 (+) human breast cancer cells. Breast Cancer Res Treat. DOI 10.1007/s10549-10011-11692-y

Curry HA, Clemens RA, Shah S, Bradbury CM, Botero A, Goswami P, Gius D (1999) Heat shock inhibits radiation-induced activation of NFkappaB via inhibition of I-kappaB kinase. J Biol Chem 274:23061–23067

Dalerba P, Cho RW, Clarke MF (2007) Cancer stem cells: models and concepts. Annu Rev Med 58:267–284

Danial NN, Korsmeyer SJ (2004) Cell death: critical control points. Cell 116:205–219

Diehn M, Cho RW, Clarke MF (2009) Therapeutic implications of the cancer stem cell hypothesis. Semin Radiat Oncol 19:78–86

Dolcet X, Llobet D, Pallares J, Matias-Guiu X (2005) NFkB in development and progression of human cancer. Virchows Arch 446:475–482

Dylla SJ, Beviglia L, Park IK, Chartier C, Raval J, Ngan L, Pickell K, Aguilar J, Lazetic S, Smith-Berdan S, Clarke MF, Hoey T, Lewicki J, Gurney AL (2008) Colorectal cancer stem cells are enriched in xenogeneic tumors following chemotherapy. PLoS ONE 3:e2428

Eccles SA (2001) The role of c-erbB-2/HER2/neu in breast cancer progression and metastasis. J Mammary Gland Biol Neoplasia 6:393–406

Fan M, Ahmed KM, Coleman MC, Spitz DR, Li JJ (2007) Nuclear factor-kappaB and manganese superoxide dismutase mediate adaptive radioresistance in low-dose irradiated mouse skin epithelial cells. Cancer Res 67:3220–3228

Feinendegen LE (1999) The role of adaptive responses following exposure to ionizing radiation. Hum Exp Toxicol 18:426–432

Feinendegen LE (2002) Reactive oxygen species in cell responses to toxic agents. Hum Exp Toxicol 21:85–90

Forrester HB, Albright N, Ling CC, Dewey WC (2000) Computerized video time-lapse analysis of apoptosis of REC:Myc cells X-irradiated in different phases of the cell cycle. Radiat Res 154:625–639

Frosina G (2009) DNA repair in normal and cancer stem cells, with special reference to the central nervous system. Curr Med Chem 16:854–866

Gilmore TD (2003) The Rel/NFkappa B/I kappa B signal transduction pathway and cancer. Cancer Treat Res 115:241–265

Ginestier C, Hur MH, Charafe-Jauffret E, Monville F, Dutcher J, Brown M, Jacquemier J, Viens P, Kleer CG, Liu S, Schott A, Hayes D, Birnbaum D, Wicha MS, Dontu G (2007) ALDH1 is a marker of normal and malignant human mammary stem cells and a predictor of poor clinical outcome. Cell Stem Cell 1:555–567

Granville DJ, Carthy CM, Jiang H, Levy JG, McManus BM, Matroule JY, Piette J, Hunt DW (2000) Nuclear factor-kappaB activation by the photochemotherapeutic agent verteporfin. Blood 95:256–262

Guo G, Yan-Sanders Y, Lyn-Cook BD, Wang T, Tamae D, Ogi J, Khaletskiy A, Li Z, Weydert C, Longmate JA, Huang T-T, Spitz DR, Oberley LW, Li JJ (2003) Manganese superoxide dismutase-mediated gene expression in radiation-induced adaptive responses. Mol Cell Biol 23:2362–2378

Guo G, Wang T, Gao Q, Tamae D, Wong P, Chen T, Chen WC, Shively JE, Wong JY, Li JJ (2004) Expression of ErbB2 enhances radiation-induced NFkappaB activation. Oncogene 23:535–545

Haffty BG, Brown F, Carter D, Flynn S (1996) Evaluation of HER-2 neu oncoprotein expression as a prognostic indicator of local recurrence in conservatively treated breast cancer: a case-control study. Int J Radiat Oncol Biol Phys 35:751–757

Hambardzumyan D, Becher OJ, Rosenblum MK, Pandolfi PP, Manova-Todorova K, Holland EC (2008) PI3 K pathway regulates survival of cancer stem cells residing in the perivascular niche following radiation in medulloblastoma in vivo. Genes Dev 22:436–448

Hicks DG, Yoder BJ, Pettay J, Swain E, Tarr S, Hartke M, Skacel M, Crowe JP, Budd GT, Tubbs RR (2005) The incidence of topoisomerase II-alpha genomic alterations in adenocarcinoma of the breast and their relationship to human epidermal growth factor receptor-2 gene amplification: a fluorescence in situ hybridization study. Hum Pathol 36:348–356

Holbro T, Beerli RR, Maurer F, Koziczak M, Barbas CF, Hynes NE (2003) The ErbB2/ErbB3 heterodimer functions as an oncogenic unit: ErbB2 requires ErbB3 to drive breast tumor cell proliferation. Proc Natl Acad Sci U S A 100:8933–8938

Hurt EM, Kawasaki BT, Klarmann GJ, Thomas SB, Farrar WL (2008) CD44+ CD24(−) prostate cells are early cancer progenitor/stem cells that provide a model for patients with poor prognosis. Br J Cancer 98:756–765

Jiang Z, Pore N, Cerniglia GJ, Mick R, Georgescu MM, Bernhard EJ, Hahn SM, Gupta AK, Maity A (2007) Phosphatase and tensin homologue deficiency in glioblastoma confers resistance to radiation and temozolomide that is reversed by the protease inhibitor nelfinavir. Cancer Res 67:4467–4473

Johannessen TC, Bjerkvig R, Tysnes BB (2008) DNA repair and cancer stem-like cells–potential partners in glioma drug resistance? Cancer Treat Rev 34:558–567

Jung M, Dritschilo A (2001) NFkappa B signaling pathway as a target for human tumor radiosensitization. Semin Radiat Oncol 11:346–351

Jung M, Zhang Y, Lee S, Dritschilo A (1995) Correction of radiation sensitivity in ataxia telangiectasia cells by a truncated I kappa B-alpha. Science 268:1619–1621

Jung M, Zhang Y, Dritschilo A (1997) Expression of a dominant negative I kappa B-alpha modulates hypersensitivity of ataxia telangiectasia fibroblasts to streptonigrin-induced apoptosis. Radiat Oncol Investig 5:265–268

Karin M (2006) NFkappaB and cancer: mechanisms and targets. Mol Carcinog 45:355–361

Kataoka Y, Murley JS, Khodarev NN, Weichselbaum RR, Grdina DJ (2002) Activation of the nuclear transcription factor kappaB (NFkappaB) and differential gene expression in U87 glioma cells after exposure to the cytoprotector amifostine. Int J Radiat Oncol Biol Phys 53:180–189

Kelsey KT, Memisoglu A, Frenkel D, Liber HL (1991) Human lymphocytes exposed to low doses of X-rays are less susceptible to radiation-induced mutagenesis. Mutat Res 263:197–201

Kim JJ, Tannock IF (2005) Repopulation of cancer cells during therapy: an important cause of treatment failure. Nat Rev Cancer 5:516–525

Korkaya H, Paulson A, Iovino F, Wicha MS (2008) HER2 regulates the mammary stem/progenitor cell population driving tumorigenesis and invasion. Oncogene 27:6120–6130

Kucharczak J, Simmons MJ, Fan Y, Gelinas C (2003) To be, or not to be: NFkappaB is the answer—role of Rel/NFkappaB in the regulation of apoptosis. Oncogene 22:8961–8982

Kurokawa H, Arteaga CL (2001) Inhibition of erbB receptor (HER) tyrosine kinases as a strategy to abrogate antiestrogen resistance in human breast cancer. Clin Cancer Res 7:4442

Lacroix M (2006) Significance, detection and markers of disseminated breast cancer cells. Endocr Relat Cancer 13:1033–1067

Lavon I, Fuchs D, Zrihan D, Efroni G, Zelikovitch B, Fellig Y, Siegal T (2007) Novel mechanism whereby nuclear factor kappaB mediates DNA damage repair through regulation of O(6)-methylguanine-DNA-methyltransferase. Cancer Res 67:8952–8959

Lenardo MJ, Baltimore D (1989) NFkappa B: a pleiotropic mediator of inducible and tissue-specific gene control. Cell 58:227–229

Li Q, Verma IM (2002) NFkappaB regulation in the immune system. Nat Rev Immunol 2:725–734

Li Z, Xia L, Lee ML, Khaletskiy A, Wang J, Wong JYC, Li JJ (2001) Effector genes altered in MCF-7 human breast cancer cells after exposure to fractionated ionizing radiation. Radiat Res 155:543–553

Li Z, Wang H, Eyler CE, Hjelmeland AB, Rich JN (2009) Turning cancer stem cells inside out: an exploration of glioma stem cell signaling pathways. J Biol Chem 284:16705–16709

Liang K, Lu Y, Jin W, Ang KK, Milas L, Fan Z (2003a) Sensitization of breast cancer cells to radiation by trastuzumab. Mol Cancer Ther 2:1113–1120

Liang K, Jin W, Knuefermann C, Schmidt M, Mills GB, Ang KK, Milas L, Fan Z (2003b) Targeting the phosphatidylinositol 3-kinase/Akt pathway for enhancing breast cancer cells to radiotherapy. Mol Cancer Ther 2:353–360

Locke JE, Bradbury CM, Wei SJ, Shah S, Rene LM, Clemens RA, Roti Roti J, Horikoshi N, Gius D (2002) Indomethacin lowers the threshold thermal exposure for hyperthermic radiosensitization and heat-shock inhibition of ionizing radiation-induced activation of NFkappaB. Int J Radiat Biol 78:493–502

Luo J-L, Kamata H, Karin M (2005) IKK/NFkappaB signaling: balancing life and death—a new approach to cancer therapy. J Clin Invest 115:2625–2632

Maity A, Kao GD, Muschel RJ, McKenna WG (1997) Potential molecular targets for manipulating the radiation response. Int J Radiat Oncol Biol Phys 37:639–653

Margison GP, Povey AC, Kaina B, Santibanez Koref MF (2003) Variability and regulation of O6-alkylguanine-DNA alkyltransferase. Carcinogenesis 24:625–635

Olayioye MA (2001) Update on HER-2 as a target for cancer therapy: intracellular signaling pathways of ErbB2/HER-2 and family members. Breast Cancer Res 3:385–389

Olivieri G, Bodycote J, Wolff S (1984) Adaptive response of human lymphocytes to low concentrations of radioactive thymidine. Science 223:594–597

Pardal R, Clarke MF, Morrison SJ (2003) Applying the principles of stem-cell biology to cancer. Nat Rev Cancer 3:895–902

Phillips TM, McBride WH, Pajonk F (2006) The response of CD24(−/low)/CD44+ breast cancer-initiating cells to radiation. J Natl Cancer Inst 98:1777–1785

Pianetti S, Arsura M, Romieu-Mourez R, Coffey RJ, Sonenshein GE (2001) Her-2/neu overexpression induces NFkappaB via a PI3-kinase/Akt pathway involving calpain-mediated degradation of IkappaB-alpha that can be inhibited by the tumor suppressor PTEN. Oncogene 20:1287–1299

Pietras RJ, Poen JC, Gallardo D, Wongvipat PN, Lee HJ, Slamon DJ (1999) Monoclonal antibody to HER-2/neureceptor modulates repair of radiation-induced DNA damage and enhances radiosensitivity of human breast cancer cells overexpressing this oncogene. Cancer Res 59:1347–1355

Prieur-Carrillo G, Chu K, Lindqvist J, Dewey WC (2003) Computerized video time-lapse (CVTL) analysis of the fate of giant cells produced by X-irradiating EJ30 human bladder carcinoma cells. Radiat Res 159:705–712

Puc J, Keniry M, Li HS, Pandita TK, Choudhury AD, Memeo L, Mansukhani M, Murty VV, Gaciong Z, Meek SE, Piwnica-Worms H, Hibshoosh H, Parsons R (2005) Lack of PTEN sequesters CHK1 and initiates genetic instability. Cancer Cell 7:193–204

Rich JN (2007) Cancer stem cells in radiation resistance. Cancer Res 67:8980–8984

Robson T, Price ME, Moore ML, Joiner MC, McKelvey-Martin VJ, McKeown SR, Hirst DG (2000) Increased repair and cell survival in cells treated with DIR1 antisense oligonucleotides: implications for induced radioresistance. Int J Radiat Biol 76:617–623

Romashkova JA, Makarov SS (1999) NFkappaB is a target of AKT in anti-apoptotic PDGF signalling. Nature 401:86–90

Schmidt-Ullrich RK, Dent P, Grant S, Mikkelsen RB, Valerie K (2000) Signal transduction and cellular radiation responses. Radiat Res 153:245–257

Sheridan C, Kishimoto H, Fuchs RK, Mehrotra S, Bhat-Nakshatri P, Turner CH, Goulet R, Badve S, Nakshatri H (2006). CD44+/CD24− breast cancer cells exhibit enhanced invasive properties: an early step necessary for metastasis. Breast Cancer Res 8:R59

Skov KA (1999) Perspectives on the adaptive response from studies on the response to low radiation doses (or to cisplatin) in mammalian cells. Hum Exp Toxicol 18:447–451

Skvortsova (2008) Intracellular signaling pathways regulating radioresistance of human prostate carcinoma cells. Proteomics 8:4521–4533

Slamon DJ, Clark GM, Wong SG, Levin WJ, Ullrich A, McGuire WL (1987) Human breast cancer: correlation of relapse and survival with amplification of the HER-2/neu oncogene. Science 235:177–182

Slamon DJ, Leyland-Jones B, Shak S, Fuchs H, Paton V, Bajamonde A, Fleming T, Eiermann W, Wolter J, Pegram M, Baselga J, Norton L (2001) Use of chemotherapy plus a monoclonal antibody against HER2 for metastatic breast cancer that overexpresses HER2. N Engl J Med 344:783–792

Soomro S, Shousha S, Taylor P, Shepard HM, Feldmann M (1991) c-erbB-2 expression in different histological types of invasive breast carcinoma. J Clin Pathol 44:211–214

Spitz DR, Azzam EI, Li JJ, Gius D (2004) Metabolic oxidation/reduction reactions and cellular responses to ionizing radiation: a unifying concept in stress response biology. Cancer Metastasis Rev 23:311–322

Stecca C, Gerber GB (1998) Adaptive response to DNA-damaging agents: a review of potential mechanisms. Biochem Pharmacol 55:941–951

Stockler M, Wilcken NR, Ghersi D, Simes RJ (2000) Systematic reviews of chemotherapy and endocrine therapy in metastatic breast cancer. Cancer Treat Rev 26:151–168

Summers RW, Maves BV, Reeves RD, Arjes LJ, Oberley LW (1989) Irradiation increases superoxide dismutase in rat intestinal smooth muscle. Free Radic Biol Med 6:261–270

Suzuki K, Kodama S, Watanabe M (1998) Suppressive effect of low-dose preirradiation on genetic instability induced by X rays in normal human embryonic cells. Radiat Res 150:656–662

Suzuki K, Kodama S, Watanabe M (2001) Extremely low-dose ionizing radiation causes activation of mitogen-activated protein kinase pathway and enhances proliferation of normal human diploid cells. Cancer Res 61:5396–5401

Tang G, Minemoto Y, Dibling B, Purcell NH, Li Z, Karin M, Lin A (2001) Inhibition of JNK activation through NFkappaB target genes. Nature 414:313–317

Uno M, Otsuki T, Kurebayashi J, Sakaguchi H, Isozaki Y, Ueki A, Yata K, Fujii T, Hiratsuka J, Akisada T, Harada T, Imajo Y (2001) Anti-HER2-antibody enhances irradiation-induced growth inhibition in head and neck carcinoma. Int J Cancer 94:474–479

Valabrega G, Montemurro F, Aglietta M (2007) Trastuzumab: mechanism of action, resistance and future perspectives in HER2-overexpressing breast cancer. Ann Oncol 18:977–984

Waldman T, Zhang Y, Dillehay L, Yu J, Kinzler K, Vogelstein B, Williams J (1997) Cell-cycle arrest versus cell death in cancer therapy. Nat Med 3:1034–1036

Warren CM, Landgraf R (2006) Signaling through ERBB receptors: multiple layers of diversity and control. Cell Signal 18:923–933

Weichselbaum RR, Hallahan D, Fuks Z, Kufe D (1994) Radiation induction of immediate early genes: effectors of the radiation-stress response. Int J Radiat Oncol Biol Phys 30:229–234

Wolff S (1989) Are radiation-induced effects hormetic? Science 245:575

Wolff S (1998) The adaptive response in radiobiology: evolving insights and implications. Environ Health Perspect 106(Suppl 1):277–283

Yang HY, Zhou BP, Hung MC, Lee MH (2000) Oncogenic signals of HER-2/neu in regulating the stability of the cyclin-dependent kinase inhibitor p27. J Biol Chem 275:24735–24739

Genetic Basis of Normal Tissue Radiosensitivity and Late Toxicity in Breast Cancer

Dhara MacDermed

Contents

Abstract

Individual variations in sensitivity to radiation toxicity are clinically important, but their genetic basis is poorly understood. Single nucleotide polymorphisms (SNPs) in many genes have been correlated to a higher risk of acute or late radiation toxicity. This chapter discusses cellular studies predictive of radiation sensitivity and studies of specific genes of interest, with a focus on breast cancer research. Radiogenomics studies of ATM, XRCC1, and TGFB1 are discussed, and other genes and SNPs associated with radiation toxicity are summarized. Recent results of the RAPPER study indicate that the candidate gene approach is inadequate to discover clinically useful indicators of radiation sensitivity. Genome-wide association studies (GWAS) and international collaborations may hold the key to future progress in this area.

1 Introduction

In the early days of radiation therapy, skin erythema was used as a measure of the radiation dose delivered. However, radiation oncologists have long noticed that normal tissue sensitivity to radiation can vary significantly between individuals. This is particularly evident in the case of breast cancer and head and neck cancer patients, where visible differences in the severity of radiation dermatitis are seen between individuals treated with the same dose of radiation. Occasionally, individuals will experience such debilitating acute toxicities, such as dermatitis with moist desquamation in large areas, that they require breaks from treatment or are unable to complete the planned treatment course. Late effects on the dermis, including fibrosis and telangiectasia, vary in severity as well. Individuals with greater inherent radiosensitivity could theoretically be more susceptible to toxicity with even more dire consequences, such as cardiac disease or second malignancies, but individuals could be susceptible to particular types of toxicity and not others. Investigations

D. MacDermed (✉)
St. Charles Cancer Treatment Center, Bend, OR, USA
e-mail: dharamac@gmail.com

J. Strauss et al. (eds.), *Breast Cancer Biology for the Radiation Oncologist*, Medical Radiology. Radiation Oncology,
DOI: 10.1007/174_2014_1045, © Springer-Verlag Berlin Heidelberg 2015
Published Online: 1 January 2015

into the differences in "radiosensitive" individuals have implicated a variety of genetic variations that may be responsible for the level of radiation toxicity seen in these patients. There are rare autosomal recessive syndromes caused by known genetic mutations, in which individuals are particularly radiosensitive, but patients with these syndromes are rarely encountered in clinical practice. These include ataxia-telangiectasia (caused by mutations in the ATM gene) and Nijmegen breakage syndrome (NBS, caused by mutations in NBS1). LIG4 syndrome (caused by mutations in the gene for DNA ligase IV) is very rare and has also been associated with radiation sensitivity (Chistiakov et al. 2009; Girard et al. 2004). Attempts have been made to develop assays that could measure or predict which individuals would be more sensitive to radiation, outside of these syndromes, but none have yet been applied regularly in clinical practice. This chapter reviews the evidence thus far on the genetic basis of normal tissue radiosensitivity, including early and late toxicity, with a focus on topics relevant to breast cancer treatment. Most of the evidence has been accumulated in the modern era of "radiogenomics", defined by Catharine West as the study of the genetic variation that underlies how a cancer patient responds to radiotherapy (West et al. 2001).

2   Cellular Studies Predictive of Radiation Sensitivity

Direct observation and measurement of radiation sensitivity in human lymphocytes and fibroblasts has supported the hypothesis that individuals vary greatly in the radiation sensitivity of their normal cells (Burnet et al. 1992). Presumably, this is due to their genomic variations and may very well represent polygenic effects. The potential of in vitro radiosensitivity to predict clinically relevant normal tissue toxicity has been demonstrated in some studies, but no individual cellular assay has been well established to determine an individual's likelihood of radiation toxicity.

Burnet and colleagues in the UK and Sweden obtained skin fibroblast lines from six patients treated with radiation after mastectomy for breast cancer. Patients were selected from a clinical trial to represent a wide range of acute and late normal tissue reactions. Radiation survival curves were generated for these fibroblast lines, and a "striking relationship" was seen between in vitro sensitivity and radiation toxicity, particularly with acute reactions (Burnet et al. 1992). Fibroblast clonogenic assays require 2–3 months to yield results and thus are not clinically useful. West and collaborators in Manchester carried out a prospective study in cervical cancer in which peripheral lymphocytes were grown from 123 patients with cervical cancer (West et al. 2001). Clonogenic assays were

carried out to determine inherent radiosensitivity. The radiosensitivity of these lymphocytes was a prognostic factor for late morbidity in pelvic organs. Unfortunately, the authors reported that the assay is not suited for clinical use, because assay errors were around one-half of the variation between individuals. Further development of predictive assays has more recently focused on specific genetic alterations, rather than an in vitro cellular phenotype.

3   BRCA1 and BRCA2 Mutations

Two genes that are mutated in familial cancer susceptibility, BRCA1 and BRCA2, are tumor suppressor genes involved in DNA damage repair and genome stabilization and thus have been suspected as factors in radiation toxicity. The normal BRCA1 and BRCA2 proteins are involved in DNA double-strand break repair by homologous recombination. Heterozygous mutations in these genes, including a variety of protein-truncating mutations, have been found in most cases of truly hereditary breast cancer. These mutations are the subject of routine testing in patients with a family history suggestive of hereditary susceptibility. Many different approaches have been taken to examine the relationship between BRCA1 and BRCA2 in radiation toxicity, and most results have been negative.

Leong and collaborators in Australia identified 22 cancer patients, 12 of whom were breast cancer patients, who developed particularly severe acute or late radiation toxicities (Leong et al. 2000). BRCA1 and BRCA2 mutations were assayed using a protein truncation test and were not detected in any of the patients tested. Thus, these genes may not be a major cause of extreme radiation hypersensitivity. Of note, 8 of the patients had specifically been tested for ATM mutations, and these were also negative.

Another approach is to take known carriers of BRCA1 and BRCA2 mutations and to measure the radiosensitivity of their normal cells at a chromosomal level. Baeyens and a team in Belgium assayed chromosomal radiosensitivity in 20 breast cancer patients with BRCA1 or BRCA2 mutations and 12 healthy mutation carriers and compared them to non-carriers with breast cancer and to healthy women (Baeyens et al. 2004). Lymphocytes were exposed to radiation and then micronuclei were scored for the G0-micronucleus assay, or they were arrested after irradiation and chromatid breaks were scored in metaphase in the G2 assay. No significant differences were seen in chromosomal radiosensitivity. Contrasting findings were reported by Ernestos and colleagues in Greece, who also used the G2 assay in lymphocyte cultures from familial breast cancer patients and compared them to cells from healthy mutation carriers and healthy controls (Ernestos et al. 2010). In this study, a higher number of chromatid breaks indicated greater radiosensitivity in BRCA1 and BRCA2 carriers, whether they were breast cancer patients or healthy carriers, compare to normal controls.

Despite the increased radiation sensitivity demonstrated by some in vitro studies (Shanley et al. 2006; Buchholz et al. 2002), multiple clinical studies have shown no impact of BRCA1 and BRCA2 mutations on the radiation toxicity observed in patients. A multicenter analysis in North America, published by Pierce, reported no difference in acute and chronic toxicity from breast cancer radiotherapy in 71 mutation carriers and matched controls at 5 years of follow-up (Pierce et al. 2000). Shanley and a large, collaborative team in the UK carried out a retrospective study of 55 BRCA1 and BRCA2 mutation carriers treated with radiation for breast cancer and compared them to matched controls with around 7 years of follow-up in both groups. There were no differences in late toxicity (Shanley et al. 2006). BRCA1 and BRCA2 mutations are thus not considered as a factor in making radiotherapy recommendations. However, these individuals are already at a higher cancer risk and may have greater chromosomal instability in response to radiation, suggesting a potentially higher risk of secondary malignancies over the long term.

4   Ataxia-Telangiectasia and the ATM Gene

The gene that has the greatest evidence linking it with normal tissue radiosensitivity in a significant number of patients is the ATM gene. Ataxia-telangiectasia, a rare autosomal recessive disease, is caused by homozygous mutations in the ATM gene. In addition to neurological and immune disorders, individuals with the disease are susceptible to cancer and have extreme skin sensitivity to ionizing radiation. Cells isolated from these individuals (lymphocytes and fibroblasts) are more sensitive to ionizing radiation as well. The gene encodes a kinase that is critical in the repair of DNA double-strand breaks induced by ionizing radiation. ATM normally signals to p53, resulting in cell cycle inhibition, but this process is impaired in the mutated kinase and therefore DNA damage does not lead to cell cycle arrest. Patients with Nijmegen breakage syndrome (NBS) also have demonstrated sensitivity to ionizing radiation. ATM phosphorylates NBS, allowing NBS to form a DNA repair complex with Rad50 and MRE11 that repairs double-strand breaks. The checkpoint response to ATM may also depend on NBS. Both ataxia-telangiectasia and Nijmegen breakage syndrome are seldom seen clinically, but they offer clues as to radiation sensitivity in the larger population.

In one early study, blood relatives of patients with ataxia-telangiectasia were identified as heterozygous for "the A-T gene" based on genetic marker analysis and 13 cases were identified, 11 of whom had their breast or chest wall irradiated. These individuals did not demonstrate increased early or late normal tissue toxicity (Weissberg et al. 1998). Multiple other studies in the late 1990s that included breast cancer patients, usually with small sample sizes, used protein truncation tests and single-strand conformation polymorphism tests to identify individuals carrying ATM mutations. These failed to demonstrate a positive association with normal tissue radiation toxicity (See Table 1).

Researchers persisted with more specific and sensitive methods to detect individuals who carry germline ATM mutations without the ataxia-telangiectasia syndrome, and the majority of modern studies from the last decade showed clinical evidence of greater radiotherapy toxicity or a positive association as part of a multi-gene profile (see Table 1). Others continued to yield negative results or were not reproducible. Studies in other diseases, including prostate cancer and lung cancer, also suggested that ATM polymorphisms have an impact on radiosensitivity in other sites of the body and thus support the potential importance of this gene in breast cancer patients. These studies are summarized, with references, in Table 1.

Considered as a body of evidence, these data suggest that one possible mechanism for heightened radiosensitivity outside of a major syndrome may be seen in carriers of mutations in proteins involved in the DNA damage response, particularly in ATM mutation carriers who do not have the clinical syndrome of ataxia-telangiectasia. The significance of ATM polymorphisms in clinical practice, together with all other polymorphisms that have been linked to radiosensitivity, was cast into doubt recently due to results of a British clinical trial (Barnett et al. 2012). The study was named the RAPPER (Radiogenomics: Assessment of Polymorphisms for Predicting the Effects of Radiotherapy) trial, and the size and scope was unprecedented in the field of radiogenomics. The details of the trial will be discussed later in this chapter, but the authors suggest that most studies in this field have yielded false-negative results due to smaller sample sizes or focused on rare variants that are too rare to be clinically significant, including studies of ATM. Thirteen ATM SNPS, including those SNPs that had been previously implicated in adverse reactions to breast radiotherapy and tag SNPS designed to represent all known variants of the gene, were studied in the RAPPER trial, and none was associated significantly with radiation toxicity. Nevertheless, the strongest association in the study of 92 SNPs was found between an ATM SNP (rs4988023, a surrogate for rs1801516) and acute bladder toxicity in prostate cancer. No SNP in ATM approached significance for late sequelae in breast cancer patients.

Of course, polygenic effects may be particularly relevant to clinical practice, possibly in combination with non-genetic factors contributing to normal tissue toxicity.

Table 1 Studies correlating ATM mutation status with radiotherapy toxicity in cancer

Cancer	Patients studied	Assay	Association	References
Breast cancer				
Breast/various	23 (16 breast)	PTT	No	Appleby et al. (1997)
Breast	15	PTT	No	Ramsay et al. (1998)
Breast/various	5	PTT	No	Clarke et al. (1998)
Breast	80	PTT	No	Shayeghi et al. (1998)
Breast/various	20	SSCP	No	Oppitz et al. (1999)
Breast	46	DHPLC	Yes, late fibrosis	Iannuzzi et al. (2002)
Breast	1,100	SSCP	No	Bremer et al. (2003)
Breast	254	PTT, RFLP, DHPLC	Positive, acute and/or late reactions (Asn1853Asn), negative (intronic SNPs)	Angèle et al. (2003)
Breast	52	SNPE	No, cosmesis	Andreassen et al. (2005)
Breast	41	DHPLC	Yes, late fibrosis	Andreassen et al. (2006a)
Breast	120	DHPLC	No, late fibrosis	Andreassen et al. (2006b)
Breast	252	DHPLC	Yes, lung/pleural late effects (Leu1420Phe, others)	Edvardsen et al. (2007)
Breast	131	DHPLC	Yes, late fibrosis (1853Asn)	Ho et al. (2007)
Breast	399	MALDI-TOF	No, acute dermatitis	Suga et al. (2007)
Breast/various	34	DHPLC, RFLP	Yes, severe late (minor allele SNPs)	Azria et al. (2008)
Breast	69	RFLP, MALDI-TOF	Only in combination with risk alleles in other genes, fibrosis	Zschenker et al. (2010)
Prostate cancer				
Prostate	17	DNA seq	Yes	Hall et al. (1998)
Prostate	37	DHPLC	Yes	Cesaretti et al. (2005)
Lung cancer				
Lung	213	RFLP	Yes (−111 A and 126713 A), pneumonitis	Zhang et al. (2010)

A portion of this material is reproduced with permission of Springer-Verlag (West et al. 2010). Associations are with skin and subcutaneous soft tissue toxicity unless otherwise stated

DHPLC denaturing high performance liquid chromatography; *DNA seq* DNA sequencing; *MALDI-TOF* mass spectrometry; *PTT* protein truncation test; *RFLP* restriction fragment length polymorphism; *SNPE* single nucleotide primer extension; *SSCP* single-strand conformation polymorphism

Polymorphisms in many other genes involved in DNA double-strand break repair and in the radiation response have been hypothesized to be likely to play an important role in radiotherapy toxicity. SNP profiles or genotypes, including ATM together with multiple genes, have been associated with radiation toxicity in smaller studies of breast cancer, head and neck and other cancers (Alsbeih et al. 2010; Azria et al. 2008). These also yielded negative results in the RAPPER study (Barnett et al. 2012).

5 XRCC1 Variants

XRCC1 is a base excision repair gene that has been implicated in radiation toxicity by several studies. It has been linked to both acute reactions and late effects in breast cancer patients treated with radiation, although negative studies have also been reported (Table 2). Andreassen and team initially showed evidence correlating an XRCC1 variant to

late fibrosis and to telangiectasia after post-mastectomy radiation in 75 patients from the Danish post-mastectomy study cohort (Andreassen et al. 2003). An Arg399Arg genotype in XRCC1 (the most common genotype, found in 51 % of patients) was associated with a higher risk of grade 3 fibrosis and a higher risk of telangiectasia. This effect was enhanced in combination with other candidate SNPs. The same team was unable to reproduce the finding of increased fibrosis risk in a larger study of 120 subjects from the same cohort (Andreassen et al. 2006a, b). Several other European studies also associated acute and late radiation reactions with specific XRCC1 polymorphisms in patient cohorts of substantial size (details and references in Table 2).

The scientific investigations into this topic with the greatest numbers of patients have been conducted in Germany. Tan and colleagues in a team led by Chang-Claude conducted a study of 446 breast cancer patients, 77 of whom developed acute toxicity from radiation for breast-conserving treatment. They selected variants in 3 candidate genes and

Table 2 Studies correlating XRCC1 variants with radiotherapy toxicity, specifically in breast cancer

Patients studied	Assay	Association of studied SNP(s) or genotypes with toxicity	References
Significant associations			
41	SNPE	Positive (Arg399Arg), late fibrosis (not telangiectasia)	Andreassen et al. (2003)
254	RT-PCR and VSRED	Positive (399Gln with 194Trp), acute and/or late	Moullan et al. (2003)
247	RFLP	Positive (399Gln with 194Cys and in a genotype with 2 others), acute and/or late	Brem et al. (2006)
446	MPA	Protective (399Gln) in normal BMI, acute	Chang-Claude et al. (2005)
167	RFLP	Positive (Arg399Gln), late telangiectasia	Giotopolous et al. (2007)
399	MALDI-TOF	Protective (genotype), acute	Suga et al. (2007)
69	RFLP and MALDI-TOF	Positive (399Arg) only in genotype of 6 genes, late	Zschenker et al. (2010)
87	SNPE and RT-PCR	Positive (Arg194Trp with Arg399Gln), acute	Mangoni et al. (2011)
No significant associations			
52	RT-PCR and SNPE	None, cosmesis	Andreassen et al. (2005)
120	RT-PCR	None, late fibrosis	Andreassen et al. (2006a, b)
409	RT-PCR	None (includes 399 and 194 alone and in a genotype with 2 others), late	Chang-Claude et al. (2009)
43	RFLP	None, acute	Sterpone et al. (2010)
57	Pyro	None, late fibrosis or fat necrosis (single fraction PBI)	Falvo et al. (2012)

Associations are with skin and subcutaneous soft tissue toxicity unless otherwise stated
BMI body mass index; *MPA* melting point analysis; *PBI* partial breast irradiation; *Pyro* pyrosequencing; *RFLP* restriction fragment length polymorphism; *RT-PCR* real-time PCR; *SNPE* single nucleotide primer extension; *VSRED* variant-specific restriction enzyme digestion

used melting point analysis to detect polymorphisms. There was no significant association overall, but a protective effect of the XRCC1 Arg399Gln allele against acute toxicity was shown only in breast cancer patients of normal weight (Tan et al. 2006). Chang-Claude and team focused on late toxicity in a subsequent study, in which they prospectively genotyped 409 breast cancer patients who received radiation after breast-conserving surgery (Chang-Claude et al. 2009). The primary technique for genotyping was real-time PCR. They selected six candidate genes with functional importance in DNA repair and two "damage response" genes and selected several candidate functional polymorphisms of these genes for genotyping, including four polymorphisms of XRCC1 (one of them was Arg399Gln). They then compared the proportion of patients with the polymorphism in the patients with telangiectasia or fibrosis versus the patients without these late effects at a median follow-up of 51 months. They did not offer a subgroup analysis based on patient weight, as in their previous study. The SNPs were not associated with late toxicity, whether alone or in combination.

Patients with cancer at other sites have been the subjects of similar studies of XRCC1 polymorphisms in recent years. For instance, XRCC1 SNPs have been correlated with radiation fibrosis after lung cancer treatment (Alsbeih et al. 2010) and with acute reactions in head and neck cancers, when two SNPs in XRCC1 are found in combination

(Pratesi et al. 2011). Once again, the clinical significance of such studies is unclear in the light of the RAPPER study results. Twelve SNPs in XRCC1 were included in the trial. As with ATM, the researchers also selected tag SNPs representing all known variants in the gene and there were no statistically significant associations with radiation toxicity (Barnett et al. 2012). However, there were SNPs that came close to significance and the authors felt warranted further study in even larger patient cohorts: These included XRCC1 SNPs rs1799782 and rs25487. They were specifically associated with altered pigmentation and telangiectasia, respectively, after breast irradiation.

6   TGFB1

Another gene that has been widely implicated in radiation toxicity is TGFB1, encoding TGF-beta, a cytokine known to stimulate a strong inflammatory response and to be involved in late radiation toxicities such as pneumonitis and fibrosis (Hall and Giaccia 2011). SNPs in the gene have been linked to radiation toxicity in the treatment of breast cancer and in other sites. Alsbeih and colleagues in Saudi Arabia demonstrated a significant association of 10Leu with soft tissue fibrosis in head and neck cancers (Alsbeih et al. 2010). In prostate cancer, TGFB1 SNPs have been correlated with

Table 3 Studies correlating TGFB1 mutation status with radiotherapy toxicity in cancer

Cancer	Patients studied	Association	References
Breast cancer			
Breast	103	Yes (10Pro and −509 T), fibrosis	Quarmby et al. (2003)
Breast	41	Yes, fibrosis (10Pro and −509 T), not telangiectasia	Andreassen et al. (2003)
Breast	52	Yes, breast appearance (10Pro and −509T)	Andreassen et al. (2005)
Breast	120	No, late fibrosis	Andreassen et al. (2006a, b)
Breast	167	Positive (−509 T), late fibrosis, not telangiectasia	Giotopolous et al. (2007)
Breast	399	No (position −509 and more), acute skin effects	Suga et al. (2007)
Breast/various	34	Yes, severe late (minor allele SNPs)	Azria et al. (2008)
Breast	778	No (codon 10 or −509)	RAPPER study early report (Barnett et al. 2010)
Breast	69	Yes (only as part of a 6-gene genotype), late fibrosis	Zschenker et al. (2010)
Prostate cancer			
Prostate	141	Yes (minor alleles in codons 10 and 25, position −509), E.D., not urinary QOL	Peters et al. (2008)
Prostate	445	No (codon 10), late effects, E.D. and QOL	Meyer et al. (2009)
Prostate	197	No (position −509), late effects	Suga et al. (2008)
Other cancers			
Cervical/endometrial	78	No, late gastrointestinal	De Ruyck et al. (2006)
Head and neck	60	Yes, late fibrosis (10Leu)	Alsbeih et al. (2010)
Lung	164	Negative, pneumonitis (10Pro is protective)	Yuan et al. (2009)
Lung	213	Positive, esophagitis (−509 T)	Zhang et al. (2010)

E.D. erectile dysfunction; *QOL* quality of life

radiation toxicity in one study (Peters et al. 2008) but other reports have been negative (see Table 3). In lung cancer, TGFB1 SNPs have been associated with pneumonitis risk (Yuan et al. 2009) and esophagitis risk (Zhang et al. 2010).

This association has also been investigated in many studies of breast cancer patients (Table 3). In a study of breast cancer patients published by Andreassen, late fibrosis risk was associated with TGFB1 alleles 509T and 10Pro (Andreassen et al. 2003) and the same group also reported a higher risk of altered breast appearance with these alleles in 26 matched case–control pairs (Andreassen et al. 2005). A subsequent, larger study by the same group failed to validate the link to radiation fibrosis (Andreassen et al. 2006a, b). Over recent years, a handful of smaller studies in breast cancer gave mixed results, and a few positive associations of TGFB1 SNPs with late effects and breast fibrosis were published (Table 3). The largest study in breast cancer, prior to work by Barnett and the RAPPER trial, was reported by Suga and colleagues in Japan, who showed no relationship with acute toxicity in 399 patients. In the RAPPER trial, this gene was a focus of careful study and was represented by tag SNPs for all variants, as with ATM and XRCC1, and no significant relationship to radiotherapy toxicity was found in breast and prostate cancer treatment (Barnett et al. 2012).

7 Other Polymorphisms Implicated in DNA Repair and Radiation Toxicity

ATM, BRCA1 and BRCA2, XRCC1, and TGFB1 are only a few representatives of a long list of genes known to be important in the radiation response and DNA damage recognition and repair. Pathways that could be involved in normal tissue radiosensitivity also include activation of cell cycle checkpoints, oxidative stress responses, inflammation, and apoptosis, among others. Many studies have been carried out looking at candidate genes from these pathways and their normal variations between individuals, particularly single nucleotide polymorphisms (SNPs), to determine if there is a link to radiation sensitivity. These studies were often limited by small sample sizes and essentially failed to yield conclusive findings. No positive associations reported have been consistently validated in subsequent studies with other patient cohorts (Alsner and Andreassen 2008) and most of these yielded no statistically significant associations with late toxicity in the RAPPER study (Barnett et al. 2012). Breast cancer patients have been the most widely studied patient group in the genetic basis of radioresponse (Parliament and Murray 2010). Table 4 summarizes a number of the genes with SNPs that have been studied in this regard.

Table 4 Various genes with SNPs studied in relationship to radiotherapy toxicity in breast cancer (excludes genes summarized separately: ATM, BRCA1, BRCA2, XRCC1, and TGFB1)

Gene/SNP	Effects studied	Significant associations?	Reference(s)
ABCA1[b]	Acute	Yes, acute (3 SNPs in 2 haplotype blocks)	Isomura et al. (2008)
APEX1[b]	Acute	Yes, 148Glu with XRCC1 399Gln in normal BMI	Chang-Claude et al. (2005)
	Acute/late mixed	None	Chang-Claude et al. (2009)
	Late	None; Yes, −509T and 10Pro (breastappearance); None (fibrosis); None	Andreassen et al. (2003, 2005, 2006b), Giotopoulos et al. (2007)
CAT, MPO[b]	Acute	Yes, MPO in women with increased BMI	Ahn et al. (2006)
	Late	None (severe)	Kuptsova et al. (2008)
CDKN1A[b]	Acute	None; None	Badie et al. (2008), Tan et al. (2006)
	Mixed acute/late	None	Chang-Claude et al. (2009)
ERCC2[b]	Acute	None	Chang-Claude et al. (2005)
GSTA1[b]	Acute	None	Ambrosone et al. (2006)
	Late	Yes (telangiectasia)	Kuptsova et al. (2008)
GSTM1, GSTT1	Acute	None; None (allele deletion)	Ambrosone et al. (2006), Mangoni et al. (2011)
	Late	None	Edvardsen et al. (2007)
GSTP1[b]	Acute	Positive (105Val)	Ambrosone et al. (2006)
	Late	Positive (105Val, pleural thickening) None (severe); Positive, only as part of a 6-gene genotype (fibrosis); Positive (Ile105Val, fibrosis and fat necrosis after SF-PBI)	Edvardsen et al. (2007), Kuptsova et al. (2008), Zschenker et al. (2010), Falvo et al. (2012)
HAP1	Late fibrosis	None	Andreassen et al. (2006b), Chang-Claude et al. (2005)
IL12RB2[b]	Acute	Yes (3 SNPs in one haplotype block)	Isomura et al. (2008)
MAD2L2[b]	Acute	Positive (allele and genotype)	Suga et al. (2007)
MC1R	Mixed acute/late	Positive (160Trp, acute)	Fogarty et al. (2010)[a]
MLH1[b], MGMT	Acute	None	Mangoni et al. (2011)
MSH2[b], MSH3	Acute	Positive (MSH2 variant) and positive (MSH3 variant)	Mangoni et al. (2011)
NBN	Acute	None	Popanda et al. (2006)
	Mixed acute/late	None	Chang-Claude et al. (2009)
NOS3[b]	Acute	Yes, in women with increased BMI	Ahn et al. (2006)
	Late (severe)	Yes, telangiectasia	Kuptsova et al. (2008)

(continued)

Table 4 (continued)

Gene/SNP	Effects studied	Significant associations?	Reference(s)
OGG1	Acute	None	Sterpone et al. (2010)
RAD21[b]	Late	Positive (minor allele)	Azria et al. (2008)[a]
RAD51	Late	None (after SF-PBI)	Falvo et al. (2012)
SOD	Late	None	Andreassen et al. (2005)
SOD2[b]	Acute	None	Ahn et al. (2006)
	Late	No (codon 26, cosmesis); Positive (16Ala for fibrosis); None (fibrosis); Positive (minor allele); None (severe); Yes, only as part of a 6-gene genotype (fibrosis)	Green et al. (2002), Andreassen et al. (2003, 2006a, b), Azria et al. (2008)[a], Kuptsova et al. (2008), Zschenker et al. (2010)
TP53[b]	Acute	Protective trend in normal BMI (72Pro); None	Tan et al. (2006), Badie et al. (2008)
	Mixed acute/late	None	Chang-Claude et al. (2009)
XPD	Acute	None (Asp312Asp, Lys751Gln)	Mangoni et al. (2011)
	Late	Yes, only as part of a 6-gene genotype (fibrosis)	Zschenker et al. (2010)
XRCC2	Acute	None	Popanda et al. (2006)
	Mixed acute/late	None (including telangiectasia)	Chang-Claude et al. (2009)
XRCC3[b]	Acute	None; None; Positive (241Met)	Popanda et al. (2006), Sterpone et al. (2010), Mangoni et al. (2011)
	Mixed acute/late	None (including telangiectasia)	Chang-Claude et al. (2009)
	Late telangiectasia/ fibrosis	Positive (Thr241Thr); None (breast appearance); None; Positive (minor allele)	Andreassen et al. (2003, 2005, 2006a, b), Azria et al. (2008)[a]
		Other genes with significant associations	
ALAD[b], BAX[b], CD44[b], COMT, LIG3[b], MAP3K7[b], MAT1A[b], NEIL3[b], NFE2L2[b], OGG1, PTTG1[b], RAD9A[b], RAD17[b], REV3L[b], SHG3L1[b], TGFB3[b], TGFBR3[b]	Acute	Positive or negative (allele, genotype and/or haplotype associated with acute dermatitis)	Suga et al. (2007)
CX3CR1, DHFR, EPHX1-alpha, MTR, MTHFR	Late	None (fibrosis, telangiectasia)	Giotopoulos et al. (2007)

SF-PBI single fraction accelerated partial breast irradiation

[a] Study included other cancer sites

[b] Gene with SNP(s) included in the RAPPER trial, no statistically significant association with acute or late radiation toxicity

8   The RAPPER Trial: The End of Radiogenomics as We Know It

The RAPPER (Radiogenomics: Assessment of Polymorphisms for Predicting the Effects of Radiotherapy) study was conducted out of multiple medical facilities in the UK, with participation by Dr. Bentzen from the University of Wisconsin (Barnett et al. 2012). Blood samples were obtained from 1,613 patients in four clinical trials. 976 of these were women with breast cancer, treated with breast conservation surgery and adjuvant radiation, most of whom (942) were enrolled in a breast IMRT trial which required that the patient's conventional treatment plan had inhomogeneities resulting in substantial high-dose "hot spots" of over 107 % of the prescribed dose. These 942 patients were randomized to conventional radiation or IMRT. 34 patients in the RAPPER trial were from a separate study of breast toxicity, all of whom were treated with breast conservation therapy. The remainder of the patients in the initial analysis (871) were from two prostate cancer trials: Patients in one trial were treated with standard-dose or escalated-dose radiation and the other treated with IMRT. Toxicity data were obtained prospectively. Acute and late toxicity and cosmesis were recorded using standardized scales. A STAT score, representing an overall assessment of late toxicity at 2 years, was calculated using a validated formula. Breast toxicity end-points included breast shrinkage, telangiectasia, breast edema, pigmentation, induration/fibrosis, breast pain, and oversensitivity. A large number of clinical covariates were recorded and included in the analysis for breast cancer patients, including age, breast size, surgical cosmesis, hot spots, and acute toxicity. Prostate cancer patients had a separate set of endpoints, including late damage to multiple organs.

46 Genes and 98 SNPs in these genes were selected using a comprehensive literature search through the end of 2009, with 66 SNPs chosen because they were specifically associated with late toxicity. Others were selected because of associations with cancer susceptibility, in vitro radiosensitivity, or other functional associations. Tag SNPs were selected to cover all variants in ATM, XRCC1, TGFB1, XRCC3, and HIF1A, due to particular interest of the researchers in these genes, three of which have been carefully profiled in this chapter. Many of the other genes with SNPs included in the trial are listed in Table 4. In addition, six specific multi-gene profiles that were previously reported to be associated with radiosensitivity were analyzed. Genotypes were analyzed from blood samples using Fluidigm dynamic arrays and the Taqman sequence detection system. 92 SNPs passed quality control measures and were included in final analysis.

With corrections for covariates and multiple comparisons, no significant p-value was obtained for an association of any single SNP with the overall late toxicity score or with specific endpoints in individual cancer types (such as telangiectasias in breast cancer). The strongest association was found between an ATM SNP (rs4988023, a surrogate for rs1801516) and acute bladder toxicity in prostate cancer.

There were a few SNPs that the authors felt warranted further study in an even larger sample size, due to borderline significance above their corrected p-value threshold. For sequelae of prostate cancer treatment, these were in the genes RAD21 (urinary incontinence), SOD2 (proctitis), and SART1 (acute bladder toxicity). For breast cancer treatment, there were two SNPs in XRCC1 with borderline significance (altered pigmentation and telangiectasia). The study is continuing with further patient accrual and analysis will be repeated after longer follow-up, when more toxicity data will be available.

This large-scale research effort with meticulous statistical analysis may change the paradigm of radiogenomics research. The majority of the studies discussed in this chapter have focused on selecting candidate genes and testing them in a population of less than 500 patients, or often less than 100 patients. This approach appears to yield results that cannot be reproduced with significance in a larger patient population or with effect sizes that are too small to detect. However, the RAPPER study focused on late radiation toxicity endpoints alone, while the results of smaller studies have suggested that acute and late radiation toxicity may differ in their relationship to genetic variants. Acute toxicity could be more closely related to some of the candidate genes than late toxicity. Also, the p-value correction for multiple comparisons was a very stringent approach, given that most of the SNPs had already been correlated with toxicity in previous studies, and thus would be less likely to randomly yield false positives. Nevertheless, the results make it seem that small studies of candidate genes will probably not yield clinically useful indicators of radiation toxicity.

9   Outlook

It might be that the biological basis of radiation toxicity is still too complex to be adequately predicted by variations in one or a small set of genes. There may be interactions between large numbers of genes and other clinical and environmental factors that all contribute to how a patient's normal tissues respond to radiation. Variations in tumor response and sensitivity to chemotherapy or hormone therapy may also contribute to late outcomes. There is great motivation to elucidate this process and to discover the key elements in it, in order to enable radiation therapy to move further into the era of personalized medicine. A Radiogenomics Consortium was established in 2009 in order to help guide further research approaches and study design in radiogenomics and to enable more large-scale trials.

Genome-wide association studies (GWAS) may be a useful approach to discovering meaningful SNPs. A small genome-wide study has been reported, looking at SNPs associated with erectile dysfunction in African–American men after prostate cancer radiotherapy (Kerns et al. 2010). This identified one statistically significant SNP, in the follicle-stimulating hormone receptor (FSHR) gene, which probably would not have been selected as a candidate gene using previous methods. The team behind the RAPPER study reports that a genome-wide analysis of specific late toxicity endpoints has been done, presumably including breast cancer patients, and the team is in the process of validation and replication. They will also perform a meta-analysis of other genome-wide studies at that time. Whether there will be SNPs with clinical relevance out of this effort remains to be seen, but is likely to yield different gene candidates.

Currently, dose prescriptions and treatment planning are carried out with no knowledge of the radiation sensitivity of a given patient's normal tissues. The same normal tissue tolerance is assumed in all patients. The study of radiogenomics offers the hope of more personalized treatment planning in the future by testing patients for their radiation sensitivity profile. This could help patients to successfully complete their prescribed treatment by reducing acute toxicities and could maximize ultimate quality of life by minimizing late effects. Clearly, more scientific progress is needed before genetic profiling of radiation sensitivity can be brought to clinical practice.

References

Ahn J, Ambrosone CB, Kanetsky PA, Tian C, Lehman TA, Kropp S, Helmbold I et al (2006) Polymorphisms in genes related to oxidative stress (CAT, MnSOD, MPO, and eNOS) and acute toxicities from radiation therapy following lumpectomy for breast cancer. Clin Cancer Res Official J Am Assoc Cancer Res 12 (23):7063–7070. doi:10.1158/1078-0432.CCR-06-0039

Alsbeih G, Al-Harbi N, Al-Hadyan K, El-Sebaie M, Al-Rajhi N (2010) Association between normal tissue complications after radiotherapy and polymorphic variations in TGFB1 and XRCC1 genes. Radiat Res 173(4):505–511. doi:10.1667/RR1769.1

Alsner J, Andreassen CN (2008) Genetic markers for prediction of normal tissue toxicity after radiotherapy. Semin Radiat Oncol 18 (2):126–135

Ambrosone CB, Tian C, Ahn J, Kropp S, Helmbold I, von Fournier D, Haase W, Sautter-Bihl ML, Wenz F, Chang-Claude J (2006) Genetic predictors of acute toxicities related to radiation therapy

following lumpectomy for breast cancer: a case-series study. Breast Cancer Res (BCR) 8(4):R40. doi:10.1186/bcr1526

Andreassen CN, Alsner J, Overgaard M, Sørensen FB, Overgaard J (2006a) Risk of radiation-induced subcutaneous fibrosis in relation to single nucleotide polymorphisms in TGFB1, SOD2, XRCC1, XRCC3, APEX and ATM—a study based on dna from formalin fixed paraffin embedded tissue samples. Int J Radiat Biol 82 (8):577–586. doi:10.1080/09553000600876637

Andreassen CN, Overgaard J, Alsner J, Overgaard M, Herskind C, Cesaretti JA, Atencio DP, Green S et al (2006b) ATM sequence variants and risk of radiation-induced subcutaneous fibrosis after postmastectomy radiotherapy. Int J Radiat Oncol Biol Phys 64 (3):776–783. doi:10.1016/j.ijrobp.2005.09.014

Andreassen CN, Alsner J, Overgaard J, Herskind C, Haviland J, Owen R, Homewood J, Bliss J, Yarnold J (2005) TGFB1 polymorphisms are associated with risk of late normal tissue complications in the breast after radiotherapy for early breast cancer. Radiother Oncol J EurSocTher Radiol Oncol 75(1):18–21. doi:10.1016/j.radonc.2004. 12.012

Andreassen CN, Alsner J, Overgaard M, Overgaard J (2003) Prediction of normal tissue radiosensitivity from polymorphisms in candidate genes. Radiother Oncol J Eur Soc Ther Radiol Oncol 69(2):127–135

Angèle S, Romestaing P, Moullan N, Vuillaume M, Chapot B, Friesen M, Jongmans W et al (2003) ATM haplotypes and cellular response to DNA damage: association with breast cancer risk and clinical radiosensitivity. Cancer Res 63(24):8717–8725

Appleby JM, Barber JB, Levine E, Varley JM, Taylor AM, Stankovic T, Heighway J, Warren C, Scott D (1997) Absence of mutations in the ATM gene in breast cancer patients with severe responses to radiotherapy. Br J Cancer 76(12):1546–1549

Azria D, Ozsahin M, Kramar A, Peters S, Atencio DP, Crompton NEA, Mornex F et al (2008) Single nucleotide polymorphisms, apoptosis, and the development of severe late adverse effects after radiotherapy. Clin Cancer Res Official J Am Assoc Cancer Res 14(19):6284–6288. doi:10.1158/1078-0432.CCR-08-0700

Badie C, Dziwura S, Raffy C, Tsigani T, Alsbeih G, Moody J, Finnon P, Levine E, Scott D, Bouffler S (2008) Aberrant CDKN1A transcriptional response associates with abnormal sensitivity to radiation treatment. Br J Cancer 98(11):1845–1851. doi:10.1038/sj. bjc.6604381

Baeyens A, Thierens H, Claes K, Poppe B, de Ridder L, Vral A (2004) Chromosomal radiosensitivity in BRCA1 and BRCA2 mutation carriers. Int J Radiat Biol 80(10):745–756

Barnett GC, Coles CE, Burnet NG, Pharoah PDP, Wilkinson J, West CML, Elliott RM, Baynes C, Dunning AM (2010) No association between SNPs regulating TGF-B1 secretion and late radiotherapy toxicity to the breast: results From the RAPPER study. Radiother Oncol J Eur Soc Ther Radiol Oncol 97(1):9–14. doi:10.1016/j. radonc.2009.12.006

Barnett GC, Coles CE, Elliott RM, Baynes C, Luccarini C, Conroy D, Wilkinson JS et al (2012) Independent validation of genes and polymorphisms reported to be associated with radiation toxicity: a prospective analysis study. Lancet Oncol 13(1):65–77. doi:10.1016/ S1470-2045(11)70302-3

Brem R, Cox DG, Chapot B, Moullan N, Romestaing P, Gérard J-P, Pisani P, Hall J (2006) The XRCC1 -77T→C variant: haplotypes, breast cancer risk, response to radiotherapy and the cellular response to DNA damage. Carcinogenesis 27(12):2469–2474. doi:10.1093/carcin/bgl114

Bremer M, Klöpper K, Yamini P, Bendix-Waltes R, Dörk T, Karstens JH (2003) Clinical radiosensitivity in breast cancer patients carrying pathogenic ATM gene mutations: no observation of increased radiation-induced acute or late effects. Radiother Oncol J Eur Soc Ther Radiol Oncol 69(2):155–160

Buchholz TA, Wu X, Hussain A, Tucker SL, Mills GB, Haffty B, Bergh S, Story M, Geara FB, Brock WA (2002) Evidence of haplotype insufficiency in human cells containing a germline mutation in BRCA1 or BRCA2. Int J Cancer J Int Du Cancer 97 (5):557–561

Burnet NG, Nyman J, Turesson I, Wurm R, Yarnold JR, Peacock JH (1992) Prediction of normal-tissue tolerance to radiotherapy from in-vitro cellular radiation sensitivity. Lancet 339(8809):1570–1571

Cesaretti JA, Stock RG, Lehrer S, Atencio DA, Bernstein JL, Stone NN, Wallenstein S et al (2005) ATM sequence variants are predictive of adverse radiotherapy response among patients treated for prostate cancer. Int J Radiat Oncol Biol Phys 61(1):196–202. doi:10.1016/j.ijrobp.2004.09.031

Chang-Claude J, Ambrosone CB, Lilla C (2009) Genetic polymorphisms in DNA repair and damage response genes and late normal tissue complications of radiotherapy for breast cancer. Br J Cancer 100(10):1680–1686

Chang-Claude J, Popanda O, Tan X-L, Kropp S, Helmbold I, von Fournier D, Haase W et al (2005) Association between polymorphisms in the DNA repair genes, XRCC1, APE1, and XPD and acute side effects of radiotherapy in breast cancer patients. Clin Cancer Res Official J Am Assoc Cancer Res 11(13):4802–4809. doi:10.1158/1078-0432.CCR-04-2657

Chistiakov DA, Voronova NV, Chistiakov AP (2009) Ligase IV syndrome. Eur J Med Genet 52(6):373–378. doi:10.1016/j.ejmg.2009.05.009

Clarke RA, Goozee GR, Birrell G, Fang ZM, Hasnain H, Lavin M, Kearsley JH (1998) Absence of ATM truncations in patients with severe acute radiation reactions. Int J Radiat Oncol Biol Phys 41 (5):1021–1027

De Ruyck K, Van Eijkeren M, Claes K, Bacher K, Vral A, De Neve W, Thierens H (2006) TGFbeta1 polymorphisms and late clinical radiosensitivity in patients treated for gynecologic tumors. Int J Radiat Oncol Biol Phys 65(4):1240–1248. doi:10.1016/j.ijrobp.2006.03.047

Edvardsen H, Tefre T, Jansen L, Vu P, Haffty BG, Fosså SD, Kristensen VN, Børresen-Dale A-L (2007) Linkage disequilibrium pattern of the ATM gene in breast cancer patients and controls; association of SNPs and haplotypes to radio-sensitivity and post-lumpectomy local recurrence. Radiat Oncol (Lond Engl) 2:25. doi:10.1186/1748-717X-2-25

Ernestos B, Nikolaos P, Koulis G, Eleni R, Konstantinos B, Alexandra G, Michael K (2010) Increased chromosomal radiosensitivity in women carrying BRCA1/BRCA2 mutations assessed with the G2 assay. Int J Radiat Oncol Biol Phys 76(4):1199–1205. doi:10.1016/j.ijrobp.2009.10.020

Falvo Elisabetta, Strigari Lidia, Citro Gennaro, Giordano Carolina, Boboc Genoveva, Fabretti Fabiana, Bruzzaniti Vicente et al (2012) SNPs in DNA repair or oxidative stress genes and late subcutaneous fibrosis in patients following single shot partial breast irradiation. J Exp Clin Cancer Res CR 31:7. doi:10.1186/1756-9966-31-7

Fogarty GB, Muddle R, Sprung CN, Chen W, Duffy D, Sturm RA, McKay MJ (2010) Unexpectedly severe acute radiotherapy side effects are associated with single nucleotide polymorphisms of the melanocortin-1 receptor. Int J Radiat Oncol Biol Phys 77(5):1486–1492

Giotopoulos G, Symonds RP, Foweraker K, Griffin M, Peat I, Osman A, Plumb M (2007) The late radiotherapy normal tissue injury phenotypes of telangiectasia, fibrosis and atrophy in breast cancer patients have distinct genotype-dependent causes. Br J Cancer 96 (6):1001–1007. doi:10.1038/sj.bjc.6603637

Girard P-M, Kysela B, Härer CJ, Doherty AJ, Jeggo PA (2004) Analysis of DNA ligase IV mutations found in LIG4 syndrome patients: the impact of two linked polymorphisms. Hum Mol Gen 13(20):2369–2376. doi:10.1093/hmg/ddh274

Green H, Ross G, Peacock J, Owen R, Yarnold J, Houlston R (2002) Variation in the manganese superoxide dismutase gene (SOD2) is not a major cause of radiotherapy complications in breast cancer patients. Radiother Oncol J Eur Soc Ther Radiol Oncol 63(2):213–216

Hall EJ, Schiff PB, Hanks GE, Brenner DJ, Russo J, Chen J, Sawant SG, Pandita TK (1998) A preliminary report: frequency of a-T heterozygotes among prostate cancer patients with severe late responses to radiation therapy. Cancer J Sci Am 4(6):385–389

Hall EJ, Giaccia A (2011) Radiobiology for the radiologist, 7th edn. Lippincott Williams & Wilkins, Philadelphia

Ho AY, Fan G, Atencio DP, Green S, Formenti SC, Haffty BG, Iyengar P et al (2007) Possession of ATM sequence variants as predictor for late normal tissue responses in breast cancer patients treated with radiotherapy. Int J Radiat Oncol Biol Phys 69(3):677–684. doi:10.1016/j.ijrobp.2007.04.012

Iannuzzi CM, Atencio DP, Green S, Stock RG, Rosenstein BS (2002) ATM mutations in female breast cancer patients predict for an increase in radiation-induced late effects. Int J Radiat Oncol Biol Phys 52(3):606–613

Isomura M, Oya N, Tachiiri S, Kaneyasu Y, Nishimura Y, Akimoto T, Hareyama M et al (2008) IL12RB2 and ABCA1 genes are associated with susceptibility to radiation dermatitis. Clin Cancer Res Official J Am Assoc Cancer Res 14(20):6683–6689. doi:10.1158/1078-0432.CCR-07-4389

Kerns SL, Ostrer H, Stock R, Li W, Moore J, Pearlman A, Campbell C et al (2010) Genome-wide association study to identify single nucleotide polymorphisms (SNPs) associated with the development of erectile dysfunction in African-American men after radiotherapy for prostate cancer. Int J Radiat Oncol Biol Phys 78(5):1292–1300. doi:10.1016/j.ijrobp.2010.07.036

Kuptsova N, Chang-Claude J, Kropp S, Helmbold I, Schmezer P, von Fournier D, Haase W et al (2008) Genetic predictors of long-term toxicities after radiation therapy for breast cancer. Int J Cancer J Int Du Cancer 122(6):1333–1339. doi:10.1002/ijc.23138

Leong T, Whitty J, Keilar M, Mifsud S, Ramsay J, Birrell G, Venter D, Southey M, McKay M (2000) Mutation analysis of BRCA1 and BRCA2 cancer predisposition genes in radiation hypersensitive cancer patients. Int J Radiat Oncol Biol Phys 48(4):959–965

Mangoni M, Bisanzi S, Carozzi F, Sani C, Biti G, Livi L, Barletta E, Costantini AS, Gorini G (2011) Association between genetic polymorphisms in the XRCC1, XRCC3, XPD, GSTM1, GSTT1, MSH2, MLH1, MSH3, and MGMT genes and radiosensitivity in breast cancer patients. Int J Radiat Oncol Biol Phys 81(1):52–58. doi:10.1016/j.ijrobp.2010.04.023

Meyer A, Dörk T, Bogdanova N, Brinkhaus M-J, Wiese B, Hagemann J, Serth J et al (2009) TGFB1 gene polymorphism Leu10Pro (C.29T>C), prostate cancer incidence and quality of life in patients treated with brachytherapy. World J Urol 27(3):371–377. doi:10.1007/s00345-008-0354-0

Moullan N, Cox DG, Angèle S, Romestaing P, Gérard J-P, Hall J (2003) Polymorphisms in the DNA repair gene XRCC1, breast cancer risk, and response to radiotherapy. Cancer epidemiology, biomarkers and prevention: a publication of the American Association for Cancer Research, Cosponsored by the American Society of Preventive Oncology 12(11):1168–1174

Oppitz U, Bernthaler U, Schindler D, Sobeck A, Hoehn H, Platzer M, Rosenthal A, Flentje M (1999) Sequence analysis of the ATM gene in 20 patients with RTOG grade 3 or 4 acute and/or late tissue radiation side effects. Int J Radiat Oncol Biol Phys 44(5):981–988

Parliament MB, Murray D (2010) Single nucleotide polymorphisms of DNA repair genes as predictors of radioresponse. Semin Radiat Oncol 20(4):232–240. doi:10.1016/j.semradonc.2010.05.003

Peters CA, Stock RG, Cesaretti JA, Atencio DP, Peters S, Burri RJ, Stone NN, Ostrer H, Rosenstein BS (2008) TGFB1 single nucleotide polymorphisms are associated with adverse quality of life in prostate cancer patients treated with radiotherapy. Int J Radiat Oncol Biol Phys 70(3):752–759. doi:10.1016/j.ijrobp.2007.05.023

Pierce LJ, Strawderman M, Narod SA, Oliviotto I, Eisen A, Dawson L, Gaffney D et al (2000) Effect of radiotherapy after breast-conserving treatment in women with breast cancer and germline BRCA1/2 mutations. J Clin Oncol Official J Am Soc Clin Oncol 18(19):3360–3369

Popanda O, Tan X-L, Ambrosone CB, Kropp S, Helmbold I, von Fournier D, Haase W et al (2006) Genetic polymorphisms in the DNA double-strand break repair genes XRCC3, XRCC2, and NBS1 are not associated with acute side effects of radiotherapy in breast cancer patients. Cancer epidemiology, biomarkers and prevention: a publication of the American Association for Cancer Research, Cosponsored by the American Society of Preventive Oncology 15 (5):1048–1050. doi:10.1158/1055-9965.EPI-06-0046

Pratesi N, Mangoni M, Mancini I, Paiar F (2011) Association between single nucleotide polymorphisms in the XRCC1 and RAD51 genes and clinical radiosensitivity in head and neck cancer. Radiother Oncol 99(3):356–361

Quarmby S, Fakhoury H, Levine E, Barber J, Wylie J, Hajeer AH, West C, Stewart A, Magee B, Kumar S (2003) Association of transforming growth factor beta-1 single nucleotide polymorphisms with radiation-induced damage to normal tissues in breast cancer patients. Int J Radiat Biol 79(2):137–143

Ramsay J, Birrell G, Lavin M (1998) Testing for mutations of the ataxia telangiectasia gene in radiosensitive breast cancer patients. Radiother Oncol J Eur Soc Ther Radiol Oncol 47(2):125–128

Shanley S, McReynolds K, Ardern-Jones A, Ahern R, Fernando I, Yarnold J, Evans G et al (2006) Late toxicity is not increased in BRCA1/BRCA2 mutation carriers undergoing breast radiotherapy in the United Kingdom. Clin Cancer Res Official J Am Assoc Cancer Res 12(23):7025–7032. doi:10.1158/1078-0432.CCR-06-1244

Shayeghi M, Seal S, Regan J, Collins N, Barfoot R, Rahman N, Ashton A et al (1998) Heterozygosity for mutations in the ataxia telangiectasia gene is not a major cause of radiotherapy complications in breast cancer patients. Br J Cancer 78(7):922–927

Sterpone S, Cornetta T, Padua L, Mastellone V, Giammarino D, Testa A, Tirindelli D, Cozzi R, Donato V (2010) DNA repair capacity and acute radiotherapy adverse effects in Italian breast cancer patients. Mutat Res 684(1–2):43–48. doi:10.1016/j.mrfmmm.2009.11.009

Suga T, Ishikawa A, Kohda M, Otsuka Y, Yamada S, Yamamoto N, Shibamoto Y et al (2007) Haplotype-based analysis of genes associated with risk of adverse skin reactions after radiotherapy in breast cancer patients. Int J Radiat Oncol Biol Phys 69(3):685–693. doi:10.1016/j.ijrobp.2007.06.021

Suga T, Iwakawa M, Tsuji H, Ishikawa H, Oda E, Noda S, Otsuka Y et al (2008) Influence of multiple genetic polymorphisms on genitourinary morbidity after carbon ion radiotherapy for prostate cancer. Int J Radiat Oncol Biol Phys 72(3):808–813. doi:10.1016/j.ijrobp.2008.01.029

Tan X-L, Popanda O, Ambrosone CB, Kropp S, Helmbold I, von Fournier D, Haase W et al (2006) Association between TP53 and P21 genetic polymorphisms and acute side effects of radiotherapy in breast cancer patients. Breast Cancer Res Treat 97(3):255–262. doi:10.1007/s10549-005-9119-2

Weissberg JB, Huang DD, Swift M (1998) Radiosensitivity of normal tissues in ataxia-telangiectasia heterozygotes. Int J Radiat Oncol Biol Phys 42(5):1133–1136

West CM, Davidson SE, Elyan SA, Valentine H, Roberts SA, Swindell R, Hunter RD (2001) Lymphocyte radiosensitivity is a significant prognostic factor for morbidity in carcinoma of the cervix. Int J Radiat Oncol Biol Phys 51(1):10–15

West CML, Barnett GC, Dunning AM, Elliott RM, Burnet NG, Newman WG (2010). In: Newman WG (ed) Pharmacogenetics: making cancer treatment safer and more effective. Springer, Netherlands, Dordrecht. doi:10.1007/978-90-481-8618-1_9

Yuan X, Liao Z, Liu Z, Wang L-E, Tucker SL, Mao L, Wang XS et al (2009) Single nucleotide polymorphism at Rs1982073:T869C of the TGFbeta 1 gene is associated with the risk of radiation pneumonitis in patients with non-small-cell lung cancer treated with definitive radiotherapy. J Clin Oncol Official J Am Soc Clin Oncol 27(20):3370–3378. doi:10.1200/JCO.2008.20.6763

Zhang L, Yang M, Bi N, Fang M, Sun T, Ji W, Tan W et al (2010) ATM polymorphisms are associated with risk of radiation-induced pneumonitis. Int J Radiat Oncol Biol Phys 77(5):1360–1368. doi:10.1016/j.ijrobp.2009.07.1675

Zschenker O, Raabe A, Boeckelmann IK, Borstelmann S, Szymczak S, Wellek S, Rades D et al (2010) Association of single nucleotide polymorphisms in ATM, GSTP1, SOD2, TGFB1, XPD and XRCC1 with clinical and cellular radiosensitivity. Radiother Oncol J Eur Soc Ther Radiol Onco 97(1):26–32. doi:10.1016/j.radonc.2010.01.016

Genetic Syndromes and Radiotherapy in Breast Cancer

Camille Green, Atif J. Khan, and Bruce G. Haffty

Contents

Abstract

In this article, the controversial issue of breast-conserving therapy (lumpectomy followed by whole breast irradiation) is reviewed. Given the relatively recent identification of the BRCA1 and BRCA2 genes in the mid-1990s, the expense associated with testing, and the inherent selection biases, the available literature has inherent limitations with relatively small patient numbers and lack of prospective randomized trials in this subset of patients. However, a number of retrospective and case–control studies have demonstrated acceptable results with breast-conserving surgery and radiation, though without active prophylactic measures to reduce secondary malignancies late local in-breast relapses and contralateral secondary breast cancer events remain an issue. Acknowledging the limitations in the available data, there does not appear to be any evidence of compromised normal tissue reactions or compromised long-term survival rates in women electing breast-conserving surgery and radiation.

1 Introduction

Pierre Paul Broca in 1866 was the first to describe a familial genetic predilection to breast cancer in the literature. In his treatise, *Traité des Tumeurs*, he was able to develop a pedigree of four generations demonstrating a heritable breast cancer pattern. Dr. Broca speculated that perhaps a "germ" leads to the inheritance of this phenotype, and he wondered why it was that the individual was normal until the day the phenotype expressed itself. The pedigree Dr. Broca described had a very high penetrance. Penetrance is the likelihood that the presence of a given allele will lead to its expression, and the frequency with which a heritable trait is manifested by individuals carrying the principal gene or genes conditioning it. Complete penetrance of an allele means the gene or genes for a trait are expressed in the entire carrier population. Incomplete penetrance means the genetic trait is

C. Green · A.J. Khan (✉) · B.G. Haffty
Department of Radiation Oncology, UMDNJ-RWJMS,
Cancer Institute of New Jersey, 195 Little Albany Street,
New Brunswick, NJ 08901, USA
e-mail: khanat@umdnj.eduatif.khan@rwjuh.edu

C. Green
e-mail: mcdonaca@umdnj.edu

B.G. Haffty
e-mail: hafftybg@umdnj.edu

J. Strauss et al. (eds.), *Breast Cancer Biology for the Radiation Oncologist*, Medical Radiology. Radiation Oncology,
DOI: 10.1007/174_2014_1046, © Springer-Verlag Berlin Heidelberg 2015
Published Online: 24 January 2015

expressed in only part of the population with the allele. The highly penetrant breast cancer susceptibility genes such as BRCA1 and BRAC2 are associated with approximately 15–20 % of familial breast cancer; carriers have a 50–80 % lifetime risk of receiving a breast cancer diagnosis. CHK2, ATM, and PALB2 are intermediate penetrance genes and are characterized by rare loss of function mutations that confer a more modest risk (RR 2–4) (Turnbull et al. 2012). Many of these mutations are due to nonsense mutations.

Tumor suppressor genes exhibit a disproportionate number of nonsense mutations, while most mutations in oncogenes are missense. A nonsense mutation is a single-nucleotide base substitution or point mutation in a sequence of DNA that encodes for a premature stop codon. For example, if an original codon is CAG but undergoes a point mutation, substituting a thymine for the original cysteine. The new codon TAG now encodes a stop codon and the resulting protein will be truncated. This in turn leads to a protein product that lacks the functionality of a normal non-mutated protein.

In humans and other organisms, it has been found that after nonsense mutations take place, a process known as nonsense-mediated mRNA decay pathway (NMD) may occur. NMD is the process by which the body degrades mRNAs which contain nonsense mutations before they are translated into truncated protein products. Nonsense mutations that undergo this mRNA decay process may come to clinical attention due to loss of NMD function (Mort et al. 2008). There are several genetic diseases where this takes place, namely in the dystrophin protein in Duchenne muscular dystrophy, in the cystic fibrosis transmembrane conductance regulator gene (CFTR) in cystic fibrosis, and with β-globin in β-thalassemia. Seventy to 80 % of BRCA1 mutations identified in families with heritable breast cancer are due to nonsense mutations, or small insertions and deletions that shift the codon reading frame, causing premature protein termination. Many of these mutations likely trigger the NMD and therefore share this process in common with other genetic diseases at the molecular level.

Interestingly enough, in cystic fibrosis, the down regulation of NMD has been taken advantage of for therapy. Due to down regulation of NMD, there is an increased number of mRNA nonsense CFTR transcripts present. In the presence of gentamicin, in vivo readthrough, or overriding of the stop codons has been shown to take place, leading to expression of full-length proteins or correction of the protein function in certain patients (Linde et al. 2007; Wilschanski et al. 2000). Much of the research targeting NMD has been done in the non-oncologic setting, with cystic fibrosis, Duchenne muscular dystrophy, and Becker muscular dystrophy and has shown promise in preliminary studies. Perhaps targeting of the nonsense-mediated decay pathway in the setting of

heritable breast cancer may lead to impactful therapeutic solutions, as 70–80 % of BRCA mutations result from premature termination codons may also be regulated by NMD (Fitzgerald et al. 1996).

1.1 BRCA-Associated Breast Cancer

Breast-conserving therapy is considered standard of care for the majority of women with early-stage breast cancer, but its appropriateness in patients with germ line mutations of BRCA1 and BRCA2 is unclear and understudied. The BRCA1/2 genes are involved in the repair of DNA damage, but their full molecular functions are not completely understood. Despite concerns of enhanced radiation sensitivity leading to radiation-induced complications in normal tissues of patients with BRCA1/2 mutations, clinical experience has not supported higher rates of normal tissue reactions or complications in BRCA carriers. Still, concerns regarding elevated risks of second breast cancers in the contralateral and conservatively treated ipsilateral breast remain. The published literature on breast-conserving management of patients with BRCA1/2 mutations is reviewed in this chapter.

2 Background of Breast-Conserving Surgery and Radiation

The treatment of breast cancer was dominated by radical mastectomy or modified radical mastectomy of the affected breast prior to the 1970s (Fisher and Anderson 1994). This consists of an *en bloc* removal of the breast, muscles of the chest wall, and contents of the axilla and was considered the most appropriate local therapy for women with early-stage breast cancers. However, the results of the National Surgical Adjuvant Breast and Bowel Project (NSABP) B-06 and other studies found equivalent survival rates among women treated with either mastectomy or breast conservation therapy (or BCT, consisting of lumpectomy followed by whole breast irradiation) (Fisher et al. 2002a; Veronesi et al. 2002). The NSABP B-06, which compared mastectomy to lumpectomy with and without radiotherapy in women with invasive carcinoma, found a 39 % local recurrence rate at 20 years with lumpectomy alone, which was decreased to 14 % with the addition of radiotherapy (Fisher et al. 2002a). Several other randomized studies demonstrated statistically equal long term survival and disease-free survival rates in patients treated with BCT compared to mastectomy (Veronesi et al. 2002; Blichert-Toft et al. 1992; Poggi et al. 2003; van Dongen et al. 2000). In addition, several randomized studies comparing lumpectomy alone to lumpectomy and radiation clearly demonstrate an approximate threefold reduction in local relapse with the use of radiation following breast-conserving surgery (Clark et al. 1996; Fisher et al. 2002b; Liljegren et al. 1999; Veronesi et al. 2001; Winzer et al. 2004). From these data, BCT became the standard of care for women with stage 0, I, and II breast cancer.

BCT involves the surgical removal of the primary tumor, evaluation of the axillary nodes, and local breast irradiation; this treatment is extremely well tolerated with minimal long-term complications and favorable cosmetic outcomes (Vrieling et al. 1999, 2000). Furthermore, BCT results in improved quality of life, body image, and sexual functioning when compared with mastectomy (Verhoef et al. 1991; Blichert-Toft 1992; Schain et al. 1994), even when compared to women who have undergone chest wall reconstructions (Schain et al. 1994; Mock 1993).

3 Breast Cancer and Second Malignancies in BRCA Carriers

Breast cancer develops in approximately 12 % of women over the course of an average life span. Although many women who develop breast cancer have a family history of breast cancer, only about 5–6 % have an identifiable and/or known inherited (germ line) mutation responsible for the phenotype. Of these, mutations in BRCA1 and BRCA2 genes represent the majority. Although the prevalence of BRCA mutations in unselected American women with breast cancer is relatively low, as many as 10–20 % of very young women with breast cancer (age less than 40) and 12–30 % of breast cancers in Ashkenazi women may be attributable to BRCA mutations (Fitzgerald et al. 1996; Abeliovich et al. 1997).

The BRCA1 and BRCA2 genes function in the repair of double-strand DNA breaks through homologous recombination between DNA strands (Venkitaraman 2002). Mutations in these genes can result in the accumulation of abnormalities and a propensity for tumorigenesis. BRCA genes are inherited in an autosomal dominant fashion with variable (but usually high) penetrance. BRCA mutations have been associated with breast cancer (roughly 50–80 % lifetime risk of breast cancer), ovarian cancer (roughly 40–50 % lifetime risk for BRCA1 and 15–25 % with BRCA2), prostate cancer, and pancreatic cancer. Typical patient characteristics of BRCA-associated breast cancer can include young age at onset and bilateral involvement. Histopathology features are often more aggressive, with higher nuclear grade, aneuploidy, and high proliferation indices; tumors with a medullary component are more common among BRCA1 carriers. Estrogen and progesterone receptors are more likely to be negative in BRCA1 carriers, but

are more likely to be positive in BRCA2 carriers. Although there are some conflicting data, BRCA1/2 carriers with breast cancer appear to have equivalent survival after therapy when compared to age and staged matched patients with sporadic disease (The Breast Cancer Linkage Consortium 1999; Ansquer et al. 1998; Robson et al. 2001, 2004; Seynaeve et al. 2004).

The risk of both contralateral primary breast cancer and ovarian cancer is substantially higher in patients with BRCA1/2 mutations than sporadic counterparts. The Breast Cancer Linkage Consortium estimated a 64 % risk of contralateral breast cancer by the age of 70 years in patients who have had BRCA1-associated breast cancer (The Breast Cancer Linkage Consortium 1999; Anglian Breast Cancer Study Group 2000). The cumulative risk of ovarian cancer in these patients was 44 % by the age of 70 years. Women with BRCA2 mutations have a risk of breast cancer similar to patients with BRCA1 mutations, but have a lower risk of ovarian cancer, with a cumulative risk of less than 10 % by the age of 70 years (The Breast Cancer Linkage Consortium 1999; Robson et al. 2001; Anglian Breast Cancer Study Group 2000).

Because BRCA-associated breast cancers typically occur in young women, a host of difficult and emotionally charged issues must be considered when formulating optimal treatment strategies for these women. Competing issues include the obvious need for curative therapy, the potential toxicities and side effects of curative options, risk reduction for future malignancies, and quality-of-life issues including body image, sexual and reproductive function, as well as cancer-related anxiety, and anxiety about transmitting the mutations to children and the potential for health insurance discrimination.

4 Breast-Conserving Surgery and Radiation in BRCA Carriers

Women with BRCA-associated breast cancer may be offered mastectomy or breast-conserving surgery as an acceptable initial local therapy of the affected side. Again, it is important to note that appropriately treated women with BRCA-associated breast cancer can generally expect disease control outcomes comparable to women without BRCA mutations (adjusting for histopathological variables, age, and stage) (Brekelmans et al. 2007; Rennert et al. 2007). Women who choose ipsilateral mastectomy often may elect to have a prophylactic contralateral mastectomy (Metcalfe et al. 2008). Prophylactic mastectomy results in a 90 % risk reduction in the incidence of contralateral breast cancer (Rebbeck et al. 2004). However, a bilateral mastectomy, even with the most advanced and skillful surgical reconstructions may be a suboptimal outcome for young women desirous of breast preservation (Brandburg et al. 2008). Whether breast conservation therapy is an appropriate option for women with known deleterious mutations in the BRCA1/2 genes is unresolved but may be a reasonable strategy for young women interested in breast conservation. Since it is unlikely that a randomized trial comparing mastectomy to breast-conserving therapy specifically in BRCA1/2 carriers will be conducted in the near future, we must rely on a handful of retrospective reports to attempt to answer this question.

Haffty et al. (2002) reported on breast conservation therapy in germ line BRCA1/2 carriers with early-onset breast cancer. One hundred and twenty-seven women diagnosed with breast cancer at age 42 years or younger agreed to undergo genetic testing, and 22 were found to have BRCA1/2 mutations. It is important to note that in this series, adjuvant tamoxifen or oophorectomy was not used in any of the patients in the carrier cohort. Patients in the genetic group were younger than sporadic patients, and this difference was significant on multivariate analysis. Treatment outcomes were compared with results from patients with sporadic disease. With a median follow-up of 12.7 years, the genetic group had a higher rate of ipsilateral (49 % vs. 21 %, $p = 0.007$) and contralateral breast events (42 % vs. 9 %, $p = 0.001$). Nine of the 11 ipsilateral breast recurrences were classified as second primary tumors, based on a difference in tumor location and/or histology. Relapse-free survival in BRCA1/2 carriers was similar to noncarriers at 5 years and then progressively declined with time. Notably, all second events in BRCA1/2 carriers were successfully salvaged, and patients remained disease-free at last follow-up.

Steinmann et al. (2001) reported on a small series of BRCA1/2 carriers where they noted an increased risk of developing local relapses, particularly in BRCA1/2 carriers with bilateral disease. Similar studies by Seyneave et al. and Robson et al. also support a slightly higher rate of late ipsilateral relapses in BRCA1/2 carriers, though these did not reach statistical significance (Seynaeve et al. 2004; Haffty et al. 2002; Pierce et al. 2006; Robson et al. 1999, 2005). Robson and colleagues retrospectively reported on 87 patients who had a history of BCT for early-stage breast cancer and deleterious mutations in BRCA 1/2. They reported an IBTR rate of 14 % at 10 years (Robson et al. 2005). The authors felt this rate was comparable to the expected IBTR rate for similar patients. This report is significantly limited by the fact that oophorectomy rates in this group were not reported; 30 % of women received tamoxifen. Median follow-up for the cohort was only 76 months.

In contrast, Kirova et al. (2005) who showed no significant increase in local relapse among 29 BRCA1 carriers compared to 107 matched familial breast cancers and 271 sporadic controls. They point out, as has been noted by

several other series, that young age, rather than BRCA1/2 status, is the more important driving factor related to local relapses. In a follow-up to the Seynaeve study, Brekelmans and colleagues at the Rotterdam Family Cancer Clinic identified three cohorts of women with heritable breast cancer: cases occurring in families with known BRCA1 mutations ($n = 223$), cases occurring in families with known BRCA2 mutations ($n = 103$), and cases occurring in families tested negative for deleterious BRCA1 and 2 mutations (Brekelmans et al. 2007). In addition, they identified a sporadic breast cancer cohort without a suggestive family history ($n = 759$). Notably, the study patients were recruited from a high-risk clinic that follows families with heritable breast cancers. Individual testing was not required and uniform in the familial cohorts. The sporadic group was also untested. The median follow-up was 4.3 years in the BRCA groups and 5.1 years in the sporadic group. Forty-five percent of patient in the heritable group had breast conservation; 55 % in the sporadic group had breast conservation. No differences in local control were detected in the heritable versus sporadic groups. The BRCA-associated groups had significantly higher rates of contralateral breast cancer; no differences were detected in breast-cancer-specific survival.

Although the high rate of local relapses and contralateral events as seen in the Haffty et al. report are cause for concern, it is likely that the use of risk reduction strategies, such as tamoxifen and/or oophorectomy, would reduce these events. Specifically, several large studies in BRCA1 or BRCA2 carriers have demonstrated that the use tamoxifen, oophorectomy, or both substantially reduce the risk of secondary breast cancers in BRCA1 and BRCA2 carriers.

This was demonstrated recently in a well-conducted study of breast-conserving surgery and radiation reported by Pierce et al. (2006). In this large collaborative effort, the investigators evaluated a total of 160 BRCA1/2 mutation carriers with breast cancer matched to 445 controls with sporadic breast cancer. Median follow-up was 7.9 years for mutation carriers and 6.7 years for controls. Although there were no significant differences in IBTR between carriers and controls (15-year estimates were 24 % for carriers and 17 % for controls (hazard ratio [HR], 1.37; $P = 0.19$). A subset analysis revealed higher rates of local relapse in those carriers who had not undergone prophylactic oophorectomy. Multivariate analyses for IBTR found BRCA1/2 mutation status to be an independent predictor of IBTR when carriers who had undergone oophorectomy were removed from analysis (HR, 1.99; $P = 0.04$); the incidence of IBTR in carriers who had undergone oophorectomy was not significantly different from that in sporadic controls ($P = 0.37$). Contralateral breast cancers were significantly more frequent in carriers versus controls, with 10- and 15-year estimates of 26 and 39 % for carriers and 3 and 7 % for controls, respectively (HR, 10.43;

$P < 0.0001$). Tamoxifen use significantly reduced the risk of contralateral breast cancers in mutation carriers (HR, 0.31; $P = 0.05$). Thus, it appears that this study confirms the findings of Haffty et al. that BRCA1/2 carriers have a higher rate of both contralateral and ipsilateral breast events, if they do not undergo specific measures to reduce the risk of subsequent breast cancers by undergoing oophorectomy and/or tamoxifen.

Finally, in a noteworthy study from Pierce et al. (2000), 71 women with BRCA-associated breast cancer were matched 1:3 to 213 sporadic controls. Conditional logistic regression was used to compare rates of complications in cases versus controls. No significant increase in acute or chronic toxicities was apparent. These data are certainly reassuring for BRCA-carrying women considering breast conservation.

5 Comparison of Breast-Conserving Surgery and Mastectomy in BRCA Carriers

As noted previously, there are no randomized comparisons of breast-conserving surgery and radiation with mastectomy specifically in BRCA carriers. However, in a separate collaborative effort, Pierce and colleagues collated data on 655 patients with known deleterious mutations in the BRCA genes, 302 of whom had breast conservation, while the balance had mastectomy (Pierce et al. 2010). The 15-year cumulative estimated risk of local events as a first failure was 23.5 % following breast conservation versus 5.5 % for mastectomy ($p < 0.0001$). 15-year rates of contralateral breast cancer were similar but were expectedly high (approximately 40 %). Most importantly, regional and distant control was similar among the two groups, as was overall survival.

6 Breast-Conserving Surgery and Partial Breast Irradiation in BRCA Carriers

To date, there are no significant studies evaluating breast-conserving surgery and partial breast irradiation. Although partial breast irradiation may be considered in selected patients following breast-conserving surgery, use of partial breast irradiation in BRCA carriers should be avoided or strictly reserved to investigational studies. The recent ASTRO consensus panel classified patients with BRCA mutations as those who should not be offered partial breast irradiation outside of the context of an investigational trial (Smith et al. 2009).

7 We Will Now Examine Some of the Intermediate to Low Penetrance Genes that Play a Role in Heritable Breast Cancer

7.1 Other Genetic Syndromes Associated with Breast Cancer

7.1.1 CHEK2

CHEK2, also known as CHK2, is the human homolog of Rad53 and Cds1. These kinases are activated in response to DNA double-strand breaks or replicative stress. CHEK2 is activated by ATM and ATR. These proteins catalyze the phosphorylation of the CHEK2-specific domain leading to its transient dimerization, leading to CHEK2 autophosphorylation and its full activation. Activated CHEK2 monomers phosphorylate numerous downstream substrates, including the p53 tumor suppressor, CDC25 family proteins, and BRCA1. This in turn activates cell cycle checkpoints and increases DNA repair efficiency. In mammalian cells, CHEK2 modulates checkpoints following ionizing radiation in an ATM-dependent manner. CHEK2 phosphorylates p53 in addition to activating CDC25A and CDC25C, which in turn initiates the G1/S, S, and G2/M checkpoints, respectively (Chehab et al. 2000; Hirao et al. 2000; Matsuoka et al. 1998; Shieh et al. 2000) (3–6). In addition, BRCA1 is phosphorylated by CHEK2 following DNA damage.

Recently, studies have shown that nonsense mutations in CHEK2, encoding the CHK2 protein, were found to predict resistance to anthracycline therapy in some tumors harboring wild-type TP53 (Bertheau et al. 2007; Kandioler-Eckersberger et al. 2000; Knappskog and Lonning 2012; Lonning 2004). Further studies must be done to confirm these results.

Nonsense mutations account for approximately 11 % of all described gene lesions causing human inherited disease and approximately 20 % of disease-associated single-base pair substitutions affecting gene-coding regions. The CHEK2-1100delC mutation encodes for a nonfunctional (or "dead") kinase. Transmission of this allele is associated with somatic loss of heterozygosity in tumor specimens (Bell et al. 2007). CHEK2-1100delC mutation is a moderate risk factor for breast cancer and perhaps prostate cancer.

In some European populations, CHEK2-1100delC is present at a frequency of 1 % and confers a RR of twofold for female breast cancer and 10-fold for bilateral breast cancer and for male breast cancer in non-BRCA1/BRCA2 linked families, as well as a twofold increased risk of developing a second breast cancer. Bell et al. compared the DNA of women with familial and sporadic breast cancers in multiple ethnic groups with controls in the same ethnic groups (Bell et al. 2007).

They also searched for new CHEK2 variant polymorphisms. They found that the 1100delC mutation was present in 0.5 % of sporadic breast cancer, 0.5 % of early-onset breast cancer, and 1 % of familial breast cancer cases. Notably, an increased prevalence of CHEK2-1100delC was detected in 1.0 % of breast cancer cases in Whites and 0.8 % of African American breast cancer cases, however, it did not reach statistical significance among Latinas and was undetectable in Japanese and native Hawaiian populations. A second recurrent CHEK2 variant, P85L was observed in African American and Ashkenazi Jewish populations. However, it did not confer an increased risk to breast cancer. Another CHEK2 mutation that has generated considerable interest is I157. It is a missense variant encoding a protein capable of phosphorylating and inactivating CDC25C leading to G2 arrest. This, however, appears to be more associated with prostate cancer (Seppala et al. 2003).

The Women's Environmental, Cancer, and Radiation Epidemiology (WECARE) study is a population-based case-controlled study to compare cases with contralateral breast cancer (CBC) to cases with unilateral breast cancer. All participants are younger than 55 and were diagnosed between 1985 and 2000 with the early-stage breast cancer without lymph node involvement. Cases were diagnosed with a second invasive primary at least 1 year after primary diagnosis. Controls are patients with unilateral breast cancer who did not develop a second primary during the study period. Broeks et al. (2004) evaluated the CHEK2 (1100delC) mutation in the WECARE study population and reported a significant interaction between CHEK2 mutation status and radiation therapy. They demonstrated an elevated risk of contralateral breast cancers in affected carriers of this gene treated with radiation for their index breast cancer.

7.1.2 ATM

ATM or ataxia-telangiectasia mutated gene is located on chromosome 11q22.3 and encodes a checkpoint kinase that plays a role in DNA repair. Homozygous mutations for this gene are linked to the rare human autosomal receive disorder called ataxia telangiectasia (Savitsky et al. 1995). A heterozygous mutation of ATM does not lead to the AT phenotype, but carriers have a twofold to fivefold risk of breast cancer (Renwick et al. 2006; Tassone et al. 2003). ATM is a part of the BRCA1-associated genome surveillance complex (BASC). This complex includes MSH2, MSH6, MLH1, BLM, the RAD50–MRE11–NSB1 complex, and the DNA replicative factor C. Members of this complex have roles in recognition of abnormal or damaged DNA. It is postulated that BASC serves as a sensor of DNA damage and as a regulator of the repair process that takes place after replication (Wang et al. 2000). Studies examining single-nucleotide polymorphisms in ATM that leads to heritable diseases have been reported (Zhao et al. 2012).

Genome-wide association studies (GWAS) allow for the identification of multiple common variants predisposing to a given disease and allow for recognition of gene–gene interactions. Through the genomic analysis of 7,325 individuals, Turnbull et al. identified some examples of gene–gene interactions in breast cancer susceptibility genes; ATM, CHEK2, BRCA1, and BRCA2. They demonstrated that the frequency of ATM mutations in BRCA-positive cases is similar to that in controls, but is significantly lower in BRCA negative cases, which were defined as familial breast cancer cases without BRCA1/2 mutations. There was a similar relationship with CHEK2_1000del C. They demonstrated that in a pathway where BRCA1 or BRCA2 are mutated, the addition of an upstream mutation, such as ATM or CHEK2, might not add anything further to the risk of breast cancer. This observation would have implications for models assessing genetic risk (Turnbull et al. 2012). There are many other GWAS looking into different areas of the genome that lead to risk for hereditable breast cancer. As many of these are preliminary studies, the genome continues to answer questions while leading to many more (Brennan et al. 2012; Long et al. 2012).

Patients with ATM homozygosity who phenotypically express ataxia-telangiectasia have been shown to have fatal and/or severe reactions to radiation therapy. In these patients, radiation should be avoided. However, current efforts to see if modulated fractionation can be used in these patients to decrease their normal tissue response, which is exquisitely sensitive to radiation, are underway. Other patients with homozygous loss of function mutations that lead to DNA-repair-defective proteins have also been found to have severe and even fatal reactions to radiation. They include Nijmegen breakage syndrome, Fanconi's anemia, and DNA 4LIG deficiency (Pollard and Gatti 2009).

There are mixed and inconsistent reports regarding the effects of radiation therapy in ATM heterozygotes. Certain sequence variants of ATM may be associated with increased fibrosis, while others have reported normal tissue toxicities (Bremer et al. 2003; Edvardsen et al. 2007; Ho et al. 2006). In a study examining women enrolled in the WECARE study, there was a small but statistically significant elevated risk of contralateral breast cancers in women exposed to radiation for a first breast cancer who carried an exceptionally uncommon ATM missense variant (Broeks et al. 2004). (31) Further studies need to be done to illuminate these genetic interactions and their impact on patient outcomes.

7.1.3 TP53

TP53, or tumor protein p53, is a tumor suppressor gene located on chromosome 17p13.1 encoding a nuclear phosphoprotein. TP53 acts as a transcription factor and is involved in the control of cell cycle progression, repair of DNA damage, genomic stability, and apoptosis. In Li–Fraumeni syndrome, TP53 is mutated. This syndrome leads to an autosomal dominant predisposition to breast cancer and other forms of cancer. Most of the mutations are point mutations that lead to defective expression. However, interestingly enough, TP53 is more commonly altered in BRCA1- and BRCA2-related breast cancer than non-BRCA2-related hereditary breast cancer (Turnbull et al. 2012). However, in BRCA1 mutation carriers, the location of these TP53 mutations does not coincide with the common sites well described in noncarriers. These BRCA1 patients typically have a better prognosis when compared to those who had mutations in conserved or structural domains. When investigated on the molecular level, these mutations were found to be frameshift, nonsense, and other mutations which lead to a truncated TP53 product. Thus, loss of p53 function appears to be important in BRCA1 tumorigenesis (Alsner et al. 2000; Chappuis et al. 2000; Holstege et al. 2009). Finally, Kulkarni and colleagues recently reported that a polymorphic variant in MDM4, a key regulator of p53, resulted in earlier onset of estrogen-receptor-negative breast cancer (Kulkarni et al. 2009).

7.1.4 RAD50

RAD50 is a highly conserved component of the MRN complex and is involved early in the detection of DSB and initial processing of DNA ends. The MRN complex or MRE11–RAD50–NSB1 complex is part of the BRCA1 associated genome surveillance complex. This complex takes part in recognition of damaged DNA and is a regulator of repair. After the acquisition of double-strand breaks, the MRN complex acts to stabilize the broken strands of DNA at the break and carry out initial processing of the free DNA ends. RAD50 is thought to approximate DNA ends together to allow for further processing. The MRN complex recruits ATM to the site of damage and aids in its activation. Then, as mentioned previously, ATM goes on to activate a number of downstream targets by phosphorylation, to aid in DNA repair. RAD50 is an essential gene. Knockout mice of the mouse homologue result in embryonic lethality and sensitivity to ionizing radiation.

Brooks et al. (2012) examined 152 SNPs from six genes (CHEK2, MRE11A, MDC1, NBN, RAD50, and TP53BP1) were genotyped in the WECARE cohort to see if any of them conferred a higher risk for CBC. The authors reported an increased risk of contralateral breast cancer in patients with a particular SNP of RAD50. These results will need to validate by other groups to affect clinical practice.

7.1.5 PALB2

PALB2 was originally identified in 2006, as a BRCA-interacting protein, crucial for BCRA2 functions. PALB2 is essential to the recruitment of RAD51 to the double-strand break point in homologous recombination repair after exposure to ionizing radiation. Recent studies also suggest that PALB2

directly binds to BRCA1 to form a BRCA1–PALB2–BRCA2 complex (Zhang et al. 2009). Germ line mutations in PALB2 have been associated with a 1 % chance of hereditary breast cancers. Tischkowitz et al. (2011) analyzed patients from the WECARE study to identify nonsense or missense mutations in PALB2 that confer risk for contralateral breast cancer. They identified 5 PALB2 truncating mutations that confer increased risk of contralateral breast cancer. Additionally, different ethnic populations have been studied for the association of PALB2 mutations and increased risk for breast cancer. Recently, two rare missense variants and one common variant were identified in 139 African American women, but did not associate with increased risk of breast cancer in this small cohort (Ding et al. 2011). PALPB2 germ line deleterious truncating mutations have been associated with breast cancer in an Italian population case—control study (Balia et al. 2010).

8 Conclusions

Although the conservative management of breast cancer in patients with BRCA1 and BRCA2 germ line mutations warrants further study, the available evidence indicates that breast-conserving therapy followed by radiation therapy is an appropriate alternative to bilateral mastectomy in early-stage breast cancer in select women desirous of breast preservation. Risk counseling will be important in this group of women. Theoretical concerns for radiation-induced complications or radiation-induced malignancies have not been demonstrated to date in the available data (Pierce et al. 2000). Although development of second primary tumors in the ipsilateral and contralateral breast remains a concern for women with intact breasts, the available evidence suggests that prophylactic oophorectomy and tamoxifen will significantly reduce the probability of these secondary events (Robson et al. 2001; Pierce et al. 2006; Narod et al. 2000; Rebbeck 2000). Prophylactic oophorectomy is even more critical in the risk reduction strategy for the development of primary tumors of the ovary. For those women considering breast-conserving surgery and radiation therapy, strategies to reduce secondary events, including prophylactic oophorectomy as soon as child-bearing issues have been addressed and resolved, with or without tamoxifen or other hormonal agents as indicated, appear to be a rational and viable option. Despite some evidence that tamoxifen reduces the risk of secondary breast cancers in patients who are carriers of BRCA1 and BRCA2 mutations, the use of tamoxifen in BRCA1 breast cancer patients who are estrogen-receptor-negative remains unresolved and controversial.

It should be emphasized that the available data evaluating outcomes in BRCA1/2 carriers, although increasing, is primarily retrospective and relatively limited. Local relapse rates in these relatively small series are often confounded by other factors which may influence local relapse, including follow-up, radiation doses and techniques, use of systemic therapy, margin status, and young age. While these studies have attempted to adjust for these factors, there remain caveats in their interpretation. Since most BRCA1/2 carriers are younger women, in addition to the risk-reducing strategies outlined above to prevent second tumors in the ipsilateral and contralateral breast, careful attention should be paid to surgical technique, margin status, radiation doses, and appropriate use of systemic therapy to minimize the risk of local relapses in these young women.

References

Abeliovich D, Kaduri L, Lerer I et al (1997) The founder mutations 185delAG and 5382insC in BRCA1 and 6174delT in BRCA2 appear in 60 percent of ovarian cancer and 30 percent of early-onset breast cancer patients among Ashkenazi Jewish women. Am J Hum Genet 60:505

Alsner J, Yilmaz M, Guldberg P, Hansen LL, Overgaard J (2000) Heterogeneity in the clinical phenotype of TP53 mutations in breast cancer patients. Clin Cancer Res 6:3923–3931

Anglian Breast Cancer Study Group (2000) Prevalence and penetrance of BRCA1 and BRCA2 mutations in a population-based series of breast cancer cases. Br J Cancer 83:1301–1308

Ansquer Y, Gautier C, Fourquet A, Asselain B, Stoppa-Lyonnet D (1998) Survival in early-onset BRCA1 breast-cancer patients. Institute Curie Breast Cancer Group. Lancet 352:541

Balia C, Sensi E, Lombardi G, Roncella M, Bevilacqua G, Caligo MA (2010) PALB2: a novel inactivating mutation in a Italian breast cancer family. Fam Cancer 9:531–536

Bell DW, Kim SH, Godwin AK et al (2007) Genetic and functional analysis of CHEK2 (CHK2) variants in multiethnic cohorts. Int J Cancer 121:2661–2667

Bertheau P, Turpin E, Rickman DS et al (2007) Exquisite sensitivity of TP53 mutant and basal breast cancers to a dose-dense epirubicin-cyclophosphamide regimen. PLoS Med 4:e90

Blichert-Toft M (1992) Breast-conserving therapy for mammary carcinoma: psychosocial aspects, indications, and limitations. Ann Med 24(6):445–451

Blichert-Toft M, Rose C, Andersen JA et al (1992) Danish randomized trial comparing breast conservation therapy with mastectomy: six years of life-table analysis. Danish breast cancer cooperative group. J Natl Cancer Inst Monogr 11:19–25

Brandburg Y, Sandelin K, Erikson S et al (2008) Psychological reactions, quality of life, and body image after bilateral prophylactic mastectomy in women at high-risk for breast cancer: a prospective 1-year follow-up study. J Clin Oncol 26:3943–3949

Brekelmans CT, Tilanus-Linthorst MM, Seynaeve C et al (2007) Tumour characteristics, survival and prognostic factors of hereditary breast cancer from BRCA2-, BRCA1- and non-BRCA1/2 families as compared to sporadic breast cancer cases. Eur J Cancer 43:867–876

Bremer M, Klopper K, Yamini P, Bendix-Waltes R, Dork T, Karstens JH (2003) Clinical radiosensitivity in breast cancer patients carrying pathogenic ATM gene mutations: no observation of increased radiation-induced acute or late effects. Radiother Oncol 69:155–160

Brennan K, Garcias-Closas M, Orr N et al (2012) Intragenic ATM methylation in peripheral blood DNA as a biomarker of breast cancer risk. Cancer Res 72(9):2304–2313

Broeks A, de Witte L, Nooijen A et al (2004) Excess risk for contralateral breast cancer in CHEK2*1100delC germline mutation carriers. Breast Cancer Res Treat 83:91–93

Brooks JD, Teraoka SN, Reiner AS et al (2012) Variants in activators and downstream targets of ATM, radiation exposure, and contralateral breast cancer risk in the WECARE study. Hum Mutat 33:158–164

Chappuis PO, Nethercot V, Foulkes WD (2000) Clinico-pathological characteristics of BRCA1- and BRCA2-related breast cancer. Semin Surg Oncol 18:287–295

Chehab NH, Malikzay A, Appel M, Halazonetis TD (2000) Chk2/hCds1 functions as a DNA damage checkpoint in G(1) by stabilizing p53. Genes Dev 14:278–288

Clark RM, Whelan T, Levine M et al (1996) Randomized clinical trial of breast irradiation following lumpectomy and axillary dissection for node-negative breast cancer: an update. Ontario clinical oncology group. J Natl Cancer Inst 88:1659–1664

Ding YC, Steele L, Chu LH et al (2011) Germline mutations in PALB2 in African-American breast cancer cases. Breast Cancer Res Treat 126:227–230

Edvardsen H, Tefre T, Jansen L et al (2007) Linkage disequilibrium pattern of the ATM gene in breast cancer patients and controls; association of SNPs and haplotypes to radio-sensitivity and post-lumpectomy local recurrence. Radiat Oncol 2:25

Fisher B, Anderson S (1994) Conservative surgery for the management of invasive and noninvasive carcinoma of the breast: NSABP trials. National surgical adjuvant breast and bowel project. World J Surg 18:63–69

Fisher B, Anderson S, Bryant J et al (2002a) Twenty-year follow-up of a randomized trial comparing total mastectomy, lumpectomy, and lumpectomy plus irradiation for the treatment of invasive breast cancer. New Engl J Med 347:1233–1241

Fisher B, Bryant J, Dignam JJ et al (2002b) Tamoxifen, radiation therapy, or both for prevention of ipsilateral breast tumor recurrence after lumpectomy in women with invasive breast cancers of one centimeter or less. J Clin Oncol 20:4141–4149

Fitzgerald M, MacDonald D, Krainer M, Additional A, Additional A, Additional A (1996) Germline BRCA1 mutations in Jewish and non-Jewish women with early-onset breast cancer. N Engl J Med 1996:143

Haffty BG, Harrold E, Khan AJ et al (2002) Outcome of conservatively managed early-onset breast cancer by BRCA1/2 status. Lancet 359:1471–1477

Hirao A, Kong YY, Matsuoka S et al (2000) DNA damage-induced activation of p53 by the checkpoint kinase Chk2. Science 287:1824–1827

Ho AY, Atencio DP, Peters S et al (2006) Genetic predictors of adverse radiotherapy effects: the gene-PARE project. Int J Radiat Oncol Biol Phys 65:646–655

Holstege H, Joosse SA, van Oostrom CT, Nederlof PM, de Vries A, Jonkers J (2009) High incidence of protein-truncating TP53 mutations in BRCA1-related breast cancer. Cancer Res 69:3625–3633

Kandioler-Eckersberger D, Ludwig C, Rudas M et al (2000) TP53 mutation and p53 overexpression for prediction of response to neoadjuvant treatment in breast cancer patients. Clin Cancer Res 6:50–56

Kirova YM, Stoppa-Lyonnet D, Savignoni A, Sigal-Zafrani B, Fabre N, Fourquet A (2005) Risk of breast cancer recurrence and contralateral breast cancer in relation to BRCA1 and BRCA2 mutation status following breast-conserving surgery and radiotherapy. Eur J Cancer 41:2304–2311

Knappskog S, Lonning PE (2012) P53 and its molecular basis to chemoresistance in breast cancer. Expert Opin Ther Targets 16 (Suppl 1):S23–S30

Kulkarni DA, Vazquez A, Haffty BG et al (2009) A polymorphic variant in human MDM4 associates with accelerated age of onset of estrogen receptor negative breast cancer. Carcinogenesis 30:1910–1915

Liljegren G, Holmberg L, Bergh J et al (1999) 10-Year results after sector resection with or without postoperative radiotherapy for stage I breast cancer: a randomized trial. J Clin Oncol 17:2326–2333

Linde L, Boelz S, Nissim-Rafinia M et al (2007) Nonsense-mediated mRNA decay affects nonsense transcript levels and governs response of cystic fibrosis patients to gentamicin. J Clin Invest 117:683–692

Long J, Cai Q, Sung H et al (2012) Genome-wide association study in East asians identifies novel susceptibility Loci for breast cancer. PLoS Genet 8:e1002532

Lonning PE (2004) Genes causing inherited cancer as beacons to identify the mechanisms of chemoresistance. Trends Mol Med 10:113–118

Matsuoka S, Huang M, Elledge SJ (1998) Linkage of ATM to cell cycle regulation by the Chk2 protein kinase. Science 282:1893–1897

Metcalfe K, Lubinski J, Ghadirian P et al (2008) Predictors of contralateral prophylactic mastectomy in women with a BRCA1 or BRCA2 mutation: the hereditary breast cancer clinical study group. J Clin Oncol 26:1093–1097

Mock V (1993) Body image in women treated for breast cancer. Nurs Res 42:153–157

Mort M, Ivanov D, Cooper DN, Chuzhanova NA (2008) A meta-analysis of nonsense mutations causing human genetic disease. Hum Mutat 29:1037–1047

Narod SA, Brunet JS, Ghadirian P et al (2000) Tamoxifen and risk of contralateral breast cancer in BRCA1 and BRCA2 mutation carriers: a case-control study. Hereditary breast cancer clinical study group. Lancet 356:1876–1881

Pierce LJ, Strawderman M, Narod SA et al (2000) Effect of radiotherapy after breast-conserving treatment in women with breast cancer and germline BRCA1/2 mutations. J Clin Oncol 18:3360–3369

Pierce LJ, Levin AM, Rebbeck TR et al (2006) Ten-year multi-institutional results of breast-conserving surgery and radiotherapy in BRCA1/2-associated stage I/II breast cancer. J Clin Oncol 24:2437–2443

Pierce LJ, Phillips KA, Griffith KA et al (2010) Local therapy in BRCA1 and BRCA2 mutation carriers with operable breast cancer: comparison of breast conservation and mastectomy. Breast Cancer Res Treat 121:389–398

Poggi MM, Danforth DN, Sciuto LC et al (2003) Eighteen-year results in the treatment of early breast carcinoma with mastectomy versus breast conservation therapy: the National cancer institute randomized trial. Cancer 98:697–702

Pollard JM, Gatti RA (2009) Clinical radiation sensitivity with DNA repair disorders: an overview. Int J Radiat Oncol Biol Phys 74:1323–1331

Rebbeck TR (2000) Prophylactic oophorectomy in BRCA1 and BRCA2 mutation carriers. J Clin Oncol 18:100S–103S

Rebbeck T, Friebel T, Lynch H et al (2004) Bilateral prophylactic mastectomy reduces breast cancer risk in BRCA1 and BRCA2 mutation carriers: the PROSE study group. J Clin Oncol 22:1055

Rennert G, Bisland-Naggan S, Barnett-Griness O et al (2007) Clinical outcomes of breast cancer in carriers of BRCA1 and BRCA2 mutations. N Engl J Med 357:115–123

Renwick A, Thompson D, Seal S et al (2006) ATM mutations that cause ataxia-telangiectasia are breast cancer susceptibility alleles. Nat Genet 38:873–875

Robson M, Levin D, Federici M et al (1999) Breast conservation therapy for invasive breast cancer in Ashkenazi women with BRCA gene founder mutations. J Natl Cancer Inst 91:2112–2117

Robson ME, Boyd J, Borgen PI, Cody HS 3rd (2001) Hereditary breast cancer. Curr Probl Surg 38:387–480

Robson ME, Chappuis PO, Satagopan J et al (2004) A combined analysis of outcome following breast cancer: differences in survival based on BRCA1/BRCA2 mutation status and administration of adjuvant treatment. Breast Cancer Res 6:R8–R17

Robson M, Svahn T, McCormick B et al (2005a) Appropriateness of breast-conserving treatment of breast carcinoma in women with germline mutations in BRCA1 or BRCA2: a clinic-based series. Cancer 103:44–51

Robson M, Svahn T, McCormick B et al (2005b) Appropriateness of breast-conserving treatment of breast carcinoma in women with germline mutations in BRCA1 or BRCA2: a clinic-based series. Cancer 103:44–51

Savitsky K, Bar-Shira A, Gilad S et al (1995) A single ataxia telangiectasia gene with a product similar to PI-3 kinase. Science 268:1749–1753

Schain W, D'Angelo T, Dunn M et al (1994) Mastectomy versus conservative surgery and radiation therapy: psychosocial consequences. Cancer 73(4):1221–1228

Seppala EH, Ikonen T, Mononen N et al (2003) CHEK2 variants associate with hereditary prostate cancer. Br J Cancer 89:1966–1970

Seynaeve C, Verhoog LC, Van De Bosch LM et al (2004) Ipsilateral breast tumour recurrence in hereditary breast cancer following breast-conserving therapy. Eur J Cancer 40:1150–1158

Shieh SY, Ahn J, Tamai K, Taya Y, Prives C (2000) The human homologs of checkpoint kinases Chk1 and Cds1 (Chk2) phosphorylate p53 at multiple DNA damage-inducible sites. Genes Dev 14:289–300

Smith BD, Arthur DW, Buchholz TA et al (2009) Accelerated partial breast irradiation consensus statement from the American Society for Radiation Oncology (ASTRO). Int J Radiat Oncol Biol Phys 74:987–1001

Steinmann D, Bremer M, Rades D et al (2001) Mutations of the BRCA1 and BRCA2 genes in patients with bilateral breast cancer. Br J Cancer 85:850–858

Tassone P, Tagliaferri P, Perricelli A et al (2003) BRCA1 expression modulates chemosensitivity of BRCA1-defective HCC1937 human breast cancer cells. Br J Cancer 88:1285–1291

The Breast Cancer Linkage Consortium (1999) BRCA2 mutation carriers. J Natl Cancer Inst 91:1310–1316

Tischkowitz M, Capanu M, Sabbaghian N et al (2011) Rare germline mutations in PALB2 and breast cancer risk: a population-based study. Hum Mutat 33:674–680

Turnbull C, Seal S, Renwick A et al (2012) Gene-gene interactions in breast cancer susceptibility. Hum Mol Genet 21:958–962

van Dongen JA, Voogd AC, Fentiman IS et al (2000) Long-term results of a randomized trial comparing breast-conserving therapy with mastectomy: European organization for research and treatment of cancer 10801 trial. J Natl Cancer Inst 92:1143–1150

Venkitaraman A (2002) Cancer susceptibility and the functions of BRCA1 and BRCA2. Cell 108:171

Verhoef L, Stalpers L, Verbeek A, Wobbes T, van Daal W (1991) Breast-conserving treatment or mastectomy in early breast cancer: a clinical decision analysis with special reference to the risk of local recurrence. Eur J Cancer 27:1132–1137

Veronesi U, Marubini E, Mariani L et al (2001) Radiotherapy after breast-conserving surgery in small breast carcinoma: long-term results of a randomized trial. Ann Oncol 12:997–1003

Veronesi U, Cascinelli N, Mariani L et al (2002) Twenty-year follow-up of a randomized study comparing breast-conserving surgery with radical mastectomy for early breast cancer. N Engl J Med 347:1227–1232

Vrieling C, Collette L, Fourquet A et al (1999) The influence of the boost in breast-conserving therapy on cosmetic outcome in the EORTC "boost versus no boost" trial. EORTC radiotherapy and breast cancer cooperative groups. European organization for research and treatment of cancer. Int J Radiat Oncol Biol Phys 45:677–685

Vrieling C, Collette L, Fourquet A et al (2000) The influence of patient, tumor and treatment factors on the cosmetic results after breast-conserving therapy in the EORTC 'boost vs. no boost' trial. EORTC radiotherapy and breast cancer cooperative groups. Radiother Oncol 55:219–232

Wang Y, Cortez D, Yazdi P, Neff N, Elledge SJ, Qin J (2000) BASC, a super complex of BRCA1-associated proteins involved in the recognition and repair of aberrant DNA structures. Genes Dev 14:927–939

Wilschanski M, Famini C, Blau H et al (2000) A pilot study of the effect of gentamicin on nasal potential difference measurements in cystic fibrosis patients carrying stop mutations. Am J Respir Crit Care Med 161:860–865

Winzer KJ, Sauer R, Sauerbrei W et al (2004) Radiation therapy after breast-conserving surgery; first results of a randomised clinical trial in patients with low risk of recurrence. Eur J Cancer 40:998–1005

Zhang F, Ma J, Wu J et al (2009) PALB2 links BRCA1 and BRCA2 in the DNA-damage response. Curr Biol 19:524–529

Zhao L, Gu A, Ji G, Zou P, Zhao P, Lu A (2012) The association between ATM IVS 22-77 T>C and cancer risk: a meta-analysis. PLoS One 7:e29479

Experimental Therapies in Breast Cancer

Bryan M. Rabatic

Contents

Abstract

Advancement of radiation-based breast cancer therapy is driven by highly strategic approaches to target diseased tissue. As a core premise, radiation therapy is designed to maximize therapeutic potential while minimizing harm to surrounding healthy tissue. Recently, advances in material design, synthesis, and characterization have lead to a surge in the number of approaches intended to shrink or eliminate the tumor burden of breast cancer. These latest advancements serve as the focus of the following chapter. While the topic is broad in nature, this review will emphasize the latest advancements in molecular-based and gene-based targeting, intralesional and intra-operative designs, and, importantly, the expanding sphere of nanomaterials. The topic of nanoscale materials will be developed to include approaches of organic-based systems, inorganic-based systems, and biological hybrid nanomaterials.

1   Introduction

Traditional approaches to breast cancer management have revolved around three well-established tenants: disease excision with surgery, local control with radiation, and cytotoxic or receptor-based systemic therapy. Often these are used in a multimodal approach; the combining of treatments is intended to increased local control, disease-free survival, and freedom from distant metastasis. However, each modality is limited by morbidity for the patient and hold the possibility of mortality.

In this context, radiation therapy (RT) for breast cancer is often heralded as the least invasive of local treatment modalities. The radiation side-effect profile for breast cancer treatment is generally recognized to include a variety of skin changes (edema, erythema, and pigmentary changes), pneumonitis, pleuritis, cardiac perfusion defects, and contribution

B.M. Rabatic (✉)
Department of Radiation Oncology,
Georgia Regents University, 821 St. Sebastian Way,
Augusta, GA 30912, USA
e-mail: bmrabatic@gmail.com

J. Strauss et al. (eds.), *Breast Cancer Biology for the Radiation Oncologist*, Medical Radiology. Radiation Oncology,
DOI: 10.1007/174_2014_1047, © Springer-Verlag Berlin Heidelberg 2015
Published Online: 23 December 2015

to the risk of lymphedema and a small risk of secondary malignancy (Perez et al. 2004). Breast conservation treatment, in combination with radiotherapy, has significantly improved morbidity outcomes, while maintaining clinically relevant disease response rates (Holli et al. 2009; Veronesi et al. 2001; Fisher et al. 2002). Hormone receptor-based adjuvant therapy has evolved to become standard-of-care treatments in suitable patients (Hughes et al. 2004; Fisher et al. 2002; Fyles et al. 2004). For appropriate patients having non-metastatic disease, the effectiveness of trimodal therapy response rates is curative and serves as the goal for future therapeutic options.

Continued optimization and evolution of radiation-based treatment strategies has been the focus since Keynes' (1937) first description of breast conserving treatment in 1937. Radiotherapy has evolved to include tangential beam, 3D plans, IMRT and tomographic techniques, intra-operative, and interstitial brachytherapy approaches (Cho et al. 2002; Keall et al. 2001; Neal et al. 1995; Oliver et al. 2007; King et al. 2000; Veronesi et al. 2001). When contemplating the sophisticated microscopic and molecular nature of neoplasm, these macroscopic techniques can be considered crude tools. The future of breast cancer treatment lies in advancement of therapies at a higher resolution: the onco-scale.

Developing new therapies and materials that function at a length scale relevant to cancer is a complex challenge. Currently, our field is upon a precipice; there is great potential for therapy advancement with new materials, but it must be furnished by multi- and inter-disciplinary approaches. This chapter will serve to highlight recent advancements among relevant therapeutic disciplines that will shape future development.

2   Molecular Approaches

From the radiation oncologist's perspective, a chemical/molecular therapy to cancer therapy is typically in the adjuvant setting (Eifel et al. 2000). The well-known and well-established protocols of sequential breast cancer treatment being surgery, adjuvant chemotherapy, and/or radiation treatment are standard approaches. Concurrent chemotherapy with radiation has been successfully used (Haffty et al. 2006) however, the additional toxicity, especially with adriamycin-based chemotherapy, has relegated the approach to occasional use (Recht 2003). Conversely, concurrent receptor (i.e., HER) and hormone treatments (i.e., tamoxifen, anastrozole, and sxemestane) are routinely given with radiation schedules (Pierce et al. 2005; Ahn et al. 2005; Harris et al. 2005).

The experimental forefront of utilizing molecular approaches with radiation treatment is quite diverse and complex. For example, radiotherapy-induced gene upregulation holds particular promise for future targeted cancer treatment advancements. Investigators have demonstrated that ionizing radiation is able to activate inherent cellular cytotoxins and immune modulators within human tumors (Hallahan et al. 1995). This "gene therapy" approach is based on the finding that tumor necrosis factor (TNF-α) is upregulated with X-ray exposure. TNF-α is thought to be cytotoxic in some tumor cells and is involved in the activation of immune response (Larrick and Wright 1990). Through activation of *Egr-1* gene with irradiation, the intra-tumor concentration of TNF-α is specifically increased. This increase is confined within the treatment volume and enhanced tumor control has been shown with in vitro models (Hallahan et al. 1995).

The above concept of using radiation to activate intra-cellular processes is fostering the design of radiation-guided drug delivery for cancer cells (Hariri et al. 2010; Lowery et al. 2011). Uniquely, a treatment strategy in this approach would offer the advantages of anatomical site/tumor specificity, as determined by the treatment field, and increased bioavailability as an effect of cellular response to irradiation. For this therapy, irradiated tumors are screened in vivo against an array of phage display peptides to isolate epitopes that selectively bind tumor cells. Hallahan and co-workers have isolated a short peptide sequence of HVGGSSV, which preferentially binds irradiated cells and has been shown to serve as a targeting mechanism. To serve as a discrete therapy, the peptide can be incorporated onto the surface of liposome drug delivery system for doxorubicin. Ultimately, this type of cellular targeting allows for the enhanced delivery of chemotherapeutic agents, increased intra-tumor concentration, and lengthened half-life to augment tumor cell apoptosis, necrosis, and reduction in cell proliferation (Lowery et al. 2011). Importantly, these effects are beyond that which would be expected from an EPR-induced effect.

In a complimentary approach to modulating gene expression in tumor cells, many researchers have targeted other upregulated proteins in cancer cells. Investigators have targeted the overexpression of the oncogene protein Bcl-2 that is associated with chemoresistance and inhibition of cell apoptosis (Reed et al. 1996; Tsujimoto 1998). Lopes de Menezes and Mayer (2002) report on a Bcl-2 antisense oligonucleotide, which is combined with doxorubicin and intended to accumulate and treat mice with breast tumor xenografts. Their investigation is unique in that they elucidate the pharmacokinetics of a targeted therapy to understand the breakdown of products and systemic accumulation, in addition to the delivery of the therapeutic to the tumor site. In similar fashion, Boucier et al. (2010) have demonstrated that silencing siRNA peptides can selectively be added to the surface of drug carriers to affect gene function. Their "nanocapsule" carriers are comprised of poly(ethylene)glycol to which peptide segments are attached. They utilize specific peptide segments that target ERα to inhibit transcription of E_2, which decreases estrogen production to deregulate cell cycle progression. Their investigation shows that delivery of mixed peptide segments that target both ERα1 and ERα2 are effective in the estrogen downregulating role. Other targets of downregulation, such as PRDM14 gene expression and PRDM14 protein synthesis have also been targeted with siRNA agents (Bedi et al. 2011). This form of gene silencing can have profound impact in future therapies, furthermore, by incorporating materials that have enhanced permeability or sequestering with irradiation, more sophisticated therapies for the radiation oncologist can be envisioned.

3 Intralesional

The drive to create an intra-lesional approach is focused on attempts to further minimize morbidity for patients. Current bi- or tri-modal techniques are sequential in practice, time consuming, and physically taxing on patients. Patients undergo a surgical procedure, lesional and peri-lesion pathology is obtained, and then, if appropriate, adjuvant radiation and/or chemotherapy are commenced. In an effort to streamline this arduous process, intraoperative approaches are being created.

A wide variety of experimental approaches have sought to increase efficiency of the overall breast cancer treatment process. For instance, the speed of obtaining surgical pathology is being targeted. In a unique example, Bickford et al. (2008, 2010) are looking at a nanotechnology-based process to better detect the hormone receptor expression of breast tissue. They utilize a biophotonic system to facilitate intraoperative tumor margin assessment ex vivo at the cellular level. In this construct, core-shell nanoparticles consisting of silica coated with gold is labeled with anti-HER2/neu fragments. When incubated with breast tissue of resected samples, they noticed enhanced receptor detection in HER-positive cells (Bickford et al. 2010). They find that the ex vivo detection limits were significantly improved (five-fold increase) while correspondingly decreasing the average detection time to 5-min. The logistical advantages of faster intra-operative detection are obvious for patient benefit, in that it improves margin determination and reduces time of an operative procedure.

A novel approach for targeting lesions is being investigated by DeNardo and co-workers, as well as, other investigators (DeNardo et al. 2011; Alexiou et al. 2010; Gruttner et al. 2007; Kim et al. 2010). Their system utilizes alternating magnetic fields (AMF) to locally heat and thereby treat tumors. In this construct, chimeric monoclonal antibodies are linked to iron oxide nanoparticles and introduced systemically. Importantly, the targeting system was found to preferentially locate to the tumor volume. Tumors receiving the bioprobes and AMF had statistically decreased tumor growth rate with a significantly increased mean time to tumor repopulation (DeNardo et al. 2011). Unique here is the applied magnetic fields serve as a form of non-ionizing radiation source to locally heat and destroy the target tissue.

In the setting of a patient requiring ionizing radiation, reducing or eliminating the need for daily visits to a treatment facility is appealing. For the radiation oncologist, therapy motivation is spurred by increasing local–regional control, decreasing morbidity, and increasing survival. Currently, brachytherapy techniques are implemented with less frequency than eternal beam modalities. A technique referred to as accelerated partial breast irradiation (APBI), in which RT is delivered only to the operative bed and not the whole breast, can be delivered by a multi-cather-based approach, or a balloon or strut device. When using a balloon approach, the implant is positioned after BCS procedure and serves to define the treatment volume. For treatment, the balloon cavity is loaded with an Iridium-192 source or an electronic X-ray generator, which delivers the prescribed dose and subsequently is removed (Dooley et al. 2011; Mehta et al. 2010; Mille et al. 2010). Overall, the technique may reduce exposure to radiation healthy tissue and body organs, such as the heart and lungs (Dickler et al. 2007; Milele et al. 2009). Additionally, APBI has demonstrated equivalent control rates to whole breast irradiation following BCS in several studies (King et al. 2000; Vinci et al. 2001; Wazer et al. 2002).

4 Nanomaterials

Nanoscience has taken aim at the disease processes of a variety of cancer sites, (Conde et al. 2011; Bhattacharyya et al. 2011; Horcajada et al. 2010; Vivero-Escoto et al. 2010; Farokhzad et al. 2006) with breast tumors serving as an important target (Rivera 2003; Steinhauser et al. 2006; Tanaka et al. 2009). Formally, nanomaterials emphasize the regime of 1–100 nm (http://nano.cancer.gov; Balogh 2010), whereby manufacturing capability is seemingly the limitation to design in this unique size range. The promise of utilizing progressively decreasing length scales has established the field of nano-medicine. This developing area of science is grounded in the unique physical properties related to the complex intermolecular, intramolecular, electron orbital states, and partitioning forces that dictate material interactions at this scale (Nel et al. 2009). For cancer pharmacology, nanoparticles can be used to both passively and actively target tumors and enhance the intracellular concentration of drugs within cancer cells (Hoffman 2008; Malam et al. 2009). Specifically for the radiation oncologist, a straightforward classification scheme of these materials can broadly organized as organic-based, inorganic-based, and hybrids.

As the above description would imply, organic nanomaterials encompass the realm of drug encapsulation by liposomes or vesicles, biodegradable and synthetic polymers, and dendrimers. In contrast, inorganic nanoparticles are typically comprised of metallic, mono-element systems (i.e., silver, gold, and platinum), metal oxides, nano-ceramics, or semiconductors (also known as "quantum dots") (Sekhon and Kamboj 2010a, b). The growing popularity of these inorganic materials is related to the unique optical, electronic and thermal properties, and high efficiency cellular uptake (Murray et al. 1995; Alivisatos 1996; Jamison et al. 2007).

A particularly inspiring area of nanoparticle-based research has been with composite systems. Often referred to as nano-bio-hybrids, these materials typically consist of an inorganic nanoparticle, of which the surface has been functionalized with a biological molecule (Jamison et al. 2007; Taylor-Pashow et al. 2010; Paunesku et al. 2003; Loo et al. 2005; Liu et al. 2009). This system architecture is inherently open to biological and synthetic variability and is designable to target the onco-scale through gene and protein interactions. Overall, nanomaterials are intended to serve multiple purposes, including delivery, silencing, radiosensitization, and radioprotection and it must be noted that materials and designs are continuously evolving. The radiation oncologist should be familiar with all of these, as they work cooperatively with our treatment modality.

4.1   Organic-Based Nanomaterials

Several institutional and clinical trials have looked at using organic molecules, either individually or as self-assembled ensembles for drug delivery (Farokhzad et al. 2006; Kievit et al. 2011; Kratz et al. 2001; Kim et al. 2004). The utility of this promising area of research is a nano-drug delivery platform, which can significantly increase circulation times and/or increase concentration within tumors. One important model that has reached clinical utility has been the Abraxane formulation of paclitaxel. This material consists of paclitaxel, which is bound to a 130 nm particle of serum albumin that acts as a carrier. Albumin increases the drug circulation time and allows for improved efficacy with reduced systemic toxicity (Milele et al. 2009; Sabbatini et al. 2004). Experimental approaches continue to evolve and include a variety of delivery systems (typically lipids, small molecule amphiphiles, polymers, or dendrimers) and are constructed to encapsulate or shield a chemotherapeutic or radiosensitizer. Importantly, approaches have also included viral, protein, and peptide-based carriers (Gradishar et al. 2005). Several decades of research has been invested to understanding how liposomal or vesicular drug delivery can be enacted to deploy their drug payloads (Gradishar et al. 2005; Cho et al. 2008). As purported by Koukourakis et al. (2010) use of liposomes

can result in highly selective localization of drugs systems within tumors, which can serve as an effective modality of treatment when chemotherapy is combined with radiotherapy (Patel et al. 1984). This concept has particular importance for radiation oncology as the radiation exposure to normal tissue within the radiation field can be reduced while maintaining high intratumor concentrations of a chemo agent (Patel et al. 1984).

4.1.1   Liposomal, Micellar, and Polymeric Systems

To improve delivery of drugs systemically, molecular therapies can be encapsulated within a self-organized assembly or covalently bound to a matrix. Liposomes represent a class of self-organizing structures, which create a spherical or colloidal particle to surround a drug agent. These systems are similar to the lipid bi-layer construct of cell membranes whereby lipids or amphiphiles organize into structures to entrap a hydrophilic drug within a central cavity. To further enhance drug delivery (passively), these systems must have high circulation lifetimes. Tailoring the size and surface modifiers of nanoparticles is pivotal for increasing circulation time, in particular by avoiding the reticulendothelial system elimination pathway. Ideally, these structures should be sized to escape capture by the macrophage and filter mechanisms of the liver and spleen (less than 100 nm) (Koukourakis et al. 2010; Wisse et al. 1996) and have a hydrophilic surface which helps evades the bodily defenses and engulfment by macrophages (Yuan et al. 1995). "Nanoformulations" of cancer drugs have already been granted FDA approval with liposomal preparations for treatment of metastatic breast cancer, and these include formulations of daunorubicin and doxorubicin (Moghimi and Szebeni 2003; Markman 2006, Rivera 2003b) and are utilized with the trade names of DaunoXome®, Myocet®, and pegylated liposomal doxorubicin Doxil® and Caelyx®. These encapsulations have been able to overcome fundamental problem of poor solubility and newer formulations are currently in clinical trials (http://clinicaltrials.gov; Hofheinz et al. 2005).

Next generation liposomal systems are also being investigated for more specific cellular interactions. These targeted therapies take advantage of upregulated cell surface and endosomal receptors (Astsaturov et al. 2007; Sini 2005). By exploiting gene expression, proteins or gene fragments can become targets for therapies. These lipid-based nanoparticles have been developed to molecularly target receptors and have tumor-specific interactions to spare the surrounding healthy tissue. In breast tumor targeting, this concept has been applied to target the Bcl-2 gene, as previously described (Lopes de Menezes 2002).

Micellar networks are based on the self-organization of amphiphilic small molecules, which assemble in water to form an encapsulating vesicle. These typically are simple surfactant molecules that aggregate in similar fashion to liposomes, to form a hydrophobic core containing the chemotherapeutic drug. Genexol®-PM (PEG-poly(D,L-lactide))-paclitaxel is a micellar formulation of the taxane which has found clinical trial success with patients having refractory malignancies (Kratz et al. 2001). Importantly, in micellar systems, as well as liposomal, the amphiphile chemical structure can be customized to include ligands for targeting purposes.

In addition to the liposomal and micellar encapsulation schemes, polymeric preparations for drug delivery are also available. In this construct, the drug is either physically entrapped within or covalently bound to a polymer matrix. These polymer trapped nanoparticles act similarly to the liposomal systems to circulate within the body, extend release half-life and take advantage of enhanced permeability and retention (EPR) effect to preferentially accumulate inside a tumor. Albumin, as discussed above, is one type of polymer–drug conjugate and is a naturally occurring material, as are constructs of chitosan and heparin (Sini et al. 2005). Drugs are also conjugated to synthetic polymers that have biodegradable characteristics to aid in their elimination. Compounds of taxol and doxorubicin have been coupled to polymers of poly-L-glutamic acid (Janes et al. 2001; Yoo et al. 1999) and N-(2-hydroxypropyl)-methacrylaminde (Yoo et al. 2000). Conjugates of PGA have shown significantly enhanced lifetimes for tumor targeting (Vasey et al. 1999). Clinical trials with polyethylene glycol (PEG) and PGA-camptothecin are now in clinical trials (Kim et al. 2004; Li 2002). Wang and coworkers have developed a polymer-based delivery of paclitaxel, which specifically targets folate receptor upregulation, in a "ChemoRad" organic nanoparticle system (Bhatt et al. 2003; Wang et al. 2010).

4.1.2 Dendrimers

A synthetic extension of polymeric systems, dendrimers are novel carrier media for an incorporated therapy agent. The surge of interest in dendrimers was marked by Tomalia's finding in the mid-1980s (Werner et al. 2011). Since then, the use and complexity of dendrimers has evolved at an impressive rate (Tomalia et al. 1985; Malik et al. 1999, 2000). The interest in dendrimers lies in that they can be synthesized with a variety of peripheral functional groups, which when combined with a hydrophobic drug, solubility and bioavailability are increased.

Khan and co-workers have been pivotal in the investigation of using dendrimers in biological systems for delivery of drugs. They have identified the biodistribution of polyamidoamine (PAMAM) dendrimers to tumor and normal tissue with in vivo studies (El-Sayed et al. 2001). Continuing with this concept, they created a novel concept referred to as systemic-targeted radiation therapy (STaRT) (Nigavekar et al. 2004). Their approach is intended to create a cell targeting "nanodevice," which is a functionalized dendrimer surface intended to be used as a platform for the detection and treatment of primary and metastatic cancers. They make use of the PAMAM dendrimer construct, which is resistant to enzymatic breakdown, non-immunogenic, highly water soluble, and is able to be eventually removed from circulation by filter organs (Nigavekar et al. 2004). The nanodevice is functionalized with an αvβ3 integrin binding cyclic-RGD (Phe(f)-Lys-Arg- Gly-Asp) epitope on the surface to aid in specificity of targeting cancer cells. They found with in vitro studies, the material was non-toxic at physiologic concentrations and the binding epitope was able to specifically target the integrin pocket.

The use of folate-targeted therapies has corresponded to the increased interest in dendrimers. While many examples exist with liposome and polymeric systems, dendrimers also serve as a platform for targeting the upregulated folate receptors. Employing PAMAM dendritic polymers acetylated with folic acid, Baker and co-workers have shown that tumors can be selectively targeted with folic acid–dendrimer–methotrexate conjugates. Importantly, they demonstrated tumor volume control at significantly lower systemic dosages than control experiments, as well as improved survivability from systemic toxicities (Lesniak et al. 2007). This is especially important in that folate receptors are frequently overexpressed in breast cancer and a targeting carrier loaded with a chemotherapeutic would result in improving therapy to the tumor site, while reducing systemic toxicities. For the radiation oncologist, one can envision using this targeted scheme to also deliver a radiosensitizer and "dose paint" the treatment field.

4.2 Inorganic-Based Nanomaterials

With high atomic number (Z) materials, there is a significant probability for X-ray photon–material interaction. The subsequent photoelectric effect of this interaction has been proven to be useful for dose enhancement with iodine and gadolinium contrast agents (Kukowska-Latallo et al. 2005; Mello et al. 1983). The interest in inorganic nanoparticles and RT increased with the discovery that gold nanoparticle can form free radicals upon gamma-irradiation (Mesa et al. 1999; Khan 2003; Robar et al. 2002). The energy imparted by photoelectric and Auger electron charge transfer is relevant in that O_2^- and OH^- species are generated at the particle surface and subsequently are involved in water lysis (Rahman et al. 2009; Kong et al. 2008). It was demonstrated that microscale gold particles when loaded into cells result in an effective dose enhancement, both in vitro and in vivo (Mello et al. 1983; Misawa and Takahashi 2011). Further studies sought to answer whether metallic nanoparticles have similar utility. Several authors have showed that gold nanoparticles (AuNP) were able to enhance radiotherapy

(Robar et al. 2002; Herold et al. 2000) and further work has showed that irradiation of gold nanoparticles contributes to enhanced cancer cell death (Hainfeld et al. 2004), specifically breast cancer cells (Rahman et al. 2009). In targeting breast cancer, Kong et al. report that small diameter AuNPs ($\sim$10.8 nm) act as a cancer cell targeting moiety and have radio-cytotoxicity effects on breast cancer cell lines (Rahman et al. 2009). Extension beyond the fundamental relationship between atomic number and radiation has lead to metal NP's being used as cell imaging, imaging platforms, anti-angiogenic materials, and nanothernostics (Liu et al. 2008; Bhirde et al. 2011; Mukerjee et al. 2005). Additionally, the surface of these nanoparticles can be modified to form electron shuttles for drugs, at which point they are considered "hybrids," which will be discussed in the next section.

4.3 Hybrid Nanomaterials

A hybrid nanomaterial is specifically designed to increase both the biological activity and response of the material. Typically, these systems are composites of a metal oxide nanoparticles (titanium, silicon, and zinc) coupled to a bio-active organic molecule (Vivero-Escoto et al. 2010; Jamison et al. 2007; Taylor-Pashow et al. 2010). The spectrum of hybrid materials can range from those that are surface modified with a cell-penetrating ligand to those in which each component has a specific physical property and, when combined, create a material with multiple unique attributes (Kim et al. 2010; Xie et al. 2010; Hariri et al. 2011). Material choice ranges from that which are selectively photoactive, promote ROS formation, or are pH sensitive. Important to the utility of these systems is the ability to incorporate into cellular machinery. Several studies have reported on the uptake of nanocomposite materials, showing that multiple mechanisms are possible routes of cellular entry. Generally, phagocytosis is the preferred mechanism of entry for the immune cell, whereas, (i) clathrin-mediated endocytosis; (ii) caveolin-mediated endocytosis; (iii) macropinocytosis; and (iv) the clathrin/caveolin-independent pathway are possible for endocyctic pathways. Additionally, passive uptake is a possible mechanism for cellular entry (Tanaka et al. 2009; Rabatic et al. 2006; Mosesson et al. 2008; Johannes and Lamaze 2002).

As previously described, multi-functionality and tissue specificity are the hallmark features for developing a hybrid system. For example, the unique attributes of dendrimer systems to deliver hydrophobic drugs systemically, along with the tunable physical properties of inorganic nanoparticles, can be combined into a dendrimer nanocomposite. These materials are organic–inorganic hybrid nanoparticles composed of organic dendrimer surrounding a small, uniform domain of inorganic atoms and are termed "composite nanodevices" (CNDs). These are functional units that utilize the dendrimer exterior to serve as a biocompatible and selective targeting carrier for the therapeutic or imaging contrast inorganic material trapped within (Kirkham and Parton 2005; Balogh et al. 2007). The advantages of this system design are numerous. The dendrimers provide a 3-dimensional system, which can interact with biological systems; using PAMAM for instance, allows for cationic, anionic, neutral, lipophilic, lipophobic, or mixed surfaces carriers. When using gold, silver, or platinum inorganic domains, the properties can be individually sized and thereby "tuned" and have optimized properties (Tomalia et al. 1985; Malik et al. 1999; Kirkham and Parton 2005). The goal of these systems is to ensure that their bio-distribution is adequate for cancer treatment. Importantly, Khan and colleagues have shown these composite nanodevices with a PAMAM-gold construct, are able to preferentially target tumors.

Interestingly, these systems can also be used in the context of brachytherapy (Pan et al. 2007). For radiation medicine, CNDs combined with a radioisotope, similar to immunoisotope therapy techniques, can selectively target particular tumors, tumor sites, and/or tumor types. Additionally, the nanocomposite can be designed to carry a number of radioisotopes. Khan and colleagues have shown that ^{198}Au can be contained within the PAMAM dendrimer network and be delivered in either a fractionated or systemic method to tumor sites in vivo. These nanocomposites, due to their smaller size, are able to overcome some of the limitation of antibody-mediated delivery schemes of radioisotopes by not being diffusion limited or antigen dependant (Pan et al. 2007). This approach serves as a proof of principle design for delivery, but also lends itself to be combined with radiation-guided or receptor-guided modalities (Khan et al. 2008).

Woloschak and coworkers have been investigating the use of metal oxide nanoparticles and their uptake within cancer cell lines, as well as their ability to serve as selective carriers for chemotherapeutics (Leuschner et al. 2006). Core-shell doxorubicin nanocarriers consisting of iron oxide central core of 2–3 nm and a titanium dioxide shell for a 6–8 nm overall diameter nanocomposite particle were surface modified with doxorubicin. These nano-hybrids were studied in vitro and shown to bypass the P-glycoprotein drug resistance mechanism of ovarian cancer cells (Green et al. 2007). This system displays the unique advantage nanomaterials provide for future therapies; they demonstrate that drug delivery to adriamycin resistant cells is possible, the nanocarrier can be further functionalized for targeted therapy, and the core-shell nanocarrier construct is also functions as a MRI modality (Arora et al. 2012).

As concern increases to limit amount of radiation exposure to healthy tissue, the use of radioprotectors has gained considerable interest. Currently, free radical scavengers (aminothiols and phosphorothioates) are being trial tested to serve as a protective agents (Wu et al. 2011; Menard et al. 2003; Small 2003); however, nanohybrid materials can also be used. Protection of healthy tissues during external beam, radioimmunotherapy, or brachytherapy techniques allows for significantly higher doses of radiation that could translate into increased treatment efficacy and safety. In this context, hybrid nanoparticles capable of resisting the damaging effects of ionizing radiation are gaining interest. Dadachova and colleagues have established that fungal-derived melanin pigment, with its conjugated π-electron system, is able to dissipate high-energy electron forces and suppress secondary ionization and free radical formation (Pamugula et al. 2005). By functionalizing 20 nm silica oxide nanoparticles with a L-DOPA melanin surface coating, they have demonstrated that bone marrow can be radioprotected during RT (Schweitzer et al. 2009). In mice, the melanin covered nanoparticles impart a protective function which results in significantly elevated WBC post-irradiation levels (Schweitzer et al. 2010).

5 Conclusions

Current experimental therapies in breast cancer treatment continue the precedent of evolving at a brisk pace and have brought new insights to the interface of materials science and RT. Although these materials are complex, the nature of these novel therapies is developing with a trend toward merging disciplines. It is evident that investigators are focusing on targeted approaches and are finding novel ways of introducing therapies to safeguard normal surrounding tissue for radiotherapy patients. From a historical perspective, a targeted strategy can be fraught with fortune and disappointment. While it may be logical to target an upregulated receptor, often, we find that cancer biology is not willing to succumb to our treatment goals. The unpredictable nature of cell biology and, more specifically, cancer biology simultaneously evades and motivates us to unlock its secrets. It is necessary to continue the evolution of interdisciplinary approaches, novel materials, and accrual of knowledge to advance breast cancer treatment strategies at the onco-scale.

References

Ahn P, Vu H, Lannin D, Obedian E, DiGiovanna M, Burtness B et al (2005) Sequence of radiotherapy with tamoxifen in conservatively managed breast cancer does not affect local relapse rates. J Clin Oncol 23(1):17–23

Alexiou C, Tietze R, Schreiber E, Jorgons R (2010) Cancer therapy with drug loaded magnetic nanoparticles-magnetic drug targeting. J Magn Magn Mater 323(10):1404–1407

Alivisatos PA (1996) Semiconductor clusters, nanocrystals, and quantum dots. Science 271:933

Arora H, Jensen M, Yuan Y, Wo A, Vogt S, Paunesku T et al (2012) Nanocarriers enhance doxorubicin uptake in drug-resistant ovarian cancer cells. Cancer Res 72(3):769–778

Astsaturov I, Cohen R, Harari P (2007) EGRF-targeting monocolonal antibodies in head and neck cancer. Curr Cancer Drug Targets 7:650–665

Balogh L (2010) Why do we have so many definitions for nanoscience and nanotechnology? Nanomed Nanotechnol Biol Med 6:397–398

Balogh L, Nigavekar S, Nair B, Lesniak W, Zhang C, Sung L (2007) Significant effect of size on the in vivo biodistribution of gold composite nanodevices in mouse tumor models. Nanomed Nanotechnol Biol Med 3:281–296

Bedi D, Musacchio T, Fagbohun O, Gillespie J, Deinnocentes P, Brid C et al (2011) Delivery of siRNA into breast cancer cells via phage fusion protein-targeted liposomes. Nanomed Nanotechnol Biol Med 7(315):323

Bhatt R, de Vries P, Tulinsky J (2003) Synthesis and in vivo antitumor activity of poly(L-glutamic acid) conjugaes of 20S-camptothecin. J Med Chem 46:190–193

Bhattacharyya S, Kudgus R, Bhattachrya R, Mukherjee P (2011) Inorganic nanoparticles in cancer therapy. Pharm Res 28:237–259

Bhirde A, Xie J, Swierczewska M, Chen M (2011) Nanoparticles for cell labeling. Nanoscale 3(142):153

Bickford L, Agollah G, Drezek R, Yu T (2008) Evaluation of immunotargeted gold nanoshells as rapid diagnostic imaging agents for HER2-overexpressing breast cancer cells: a time-based analysis. Nanobiotechnology 4:1–8

Bickford L, Agollah G, Drezek R, Yu T (2010) Silica-gold nanoshells as potential intraoperative molecular probes for HER2-overexpression in ex vivo breast tissue using near-infrared confocal microscopy. Breast Cancer Res Treat 120:547–555

Bouclier C, Marsaud V, Bawa O, Nicolas V, Moine L (2010) Coadministration of nanosystems of short silencing RNAs targeting oestrogen receptor α and anti-oestrogen synergistically induces tumour growth inhibition in human breast cancer xenografts. Breast Cancer Res Treat 122:145–158

Cho B, Hurkman C, Damen E (2002) Intensity modulated versus non-intensity modulated radiotherapy in the treatment of the left breast and upper internal mammary lymph node chain: a comparative planning study. Radiother Oncol 62:127–136

Cho K, Wang X, Nie S (2008) Therapeutic nanoparticles for drug delivery in cancer. Clin Cancer Res 14:1310–1316

Conde J, Doria G, Baptista P (2011) Noble metal nanoparticles applications in cancer. J Drug Deliv 2012: in press

de Lopes Menezes D, Mayer L (2002) Pharmacokinetics of Bcl-2 antisense oligonuclieotide (GS3139) combined with doxorubicin in scid mice bearing human breast cancer solid tumor xenografts. Cancer Chemother Pharmacol 49:57–68

DeNardo S, DeNardo G, Miers L, Natarajan A, Foreman A (2011) Development of tumor targeting bioprobes (111-In chimeric l6 monoclonal antibody nanoparticles) for alternating magnetic field cancer therapy. Clin Cancer Res 11:7087s–7092s

Dickler A, Kirk M, Seif N (2007) A dosimetric comparison of mammosite high-dose-rate brachytherapy and xoft axxent electronic brachytherapy. Brachytherapy 6(2):164–168

Dooley W, Wurzer J, Megahy M, Schreiber G, Roy T, Prouix G (2011) Electronic brachytherapy as adjuvant therapy for early stage breast cancer: a retrospective analysis. OncoTargets Ther 4:13–20

Eifel P, Axelson J, Costa J, Crowley J, Curran W (2000) National institutes of health consensus development conference statement: adjuvant therapy for breast cancer. J Nat Cancer Inst 93(13):979–989

El-Sayed M, Kiani M, Naimark M, Hikal A, Ghandehari H (2001) Extravasation of poly(amidoamine) (PAMAM) dendrimers across microvascular network endothelium. Pharm Res 18:23–28

Farokhzad O, Chenng J, Telpy B, Sherifi I, Jon S, Kantoff P et al (2006) Targeted Nanoparticle-aptamer bioconjugates for cancer chemotherapy in vivo. Proc Nat Acad Sci 103(16):16315–16320

Fisher B, Anderson S, Bryant J (2002a) Twenty-year follow-up of a randomized trial comparing total mastectomy, lumpectomy, and lumpectomy plus irradiation for the treatment of invasive breast cancer. N Engl J Med 347:1233–1241

Fisher B, Bryant J, Dignam J (2002b) Tamoxifen, radiation therapy, or both for prevention of ipsilateral breast tumor recurrence after lumpectomy in women with invasive breast cancers of one centimeter or less. J Clin Oncol 20(20):4141–4149

Fyles A, McCready D, Manchul L (2004) Tamoxifen with or without breast irradiation in women 50 years of age or older with early stage breast cancer. N Engl J Med 351:963–970

Gradishar W, Tjulandin S, Davidson N (2005) Phase III trial of nanoparticle albumin-bound paclitaxel compared with polyethylated castor oil-based paclitaxel in women with breast cancer. J Clin Oncol 23:7794–7803

Green J, Chiu E, Leschiner E, Langer R, Anderson D (2007) Electrostatic ligand coatings of nanoparticles enable ligand-specific gene delivery to human primary cells. Nano Lett 7:874–879

Gruttner C, Muller K, Westphal F, Foreman A, Ivkov R (2007) Synthesis and antibody conjugation of magnetic nanoparticles with improved specific power absorption rates for alternating magnetic field cancer therapy. J Magn Magn Mater 311(1):181–186

Haffty B, Kim J, Yang Q, Higgins S (2006) Concurrent chemoradiation in the conservative management of breast cancer. Int J Radiat Oncol Biol Phys 66(5):1306–1312

Hainfeld J, Slatkin D, Smilowitz H (2004) The use of gold nanoparticles to enhance radiotherarpy in mice. Phys Med Biol 49:309–315

Hallahan D, Mauceri H, Seung L, Dunphy E, Wayne J, Hanna N et al (1995) Spatial and temporal control of gene therapy using ionizing radiation. Nat Med 1(8):786–791

Hariri G, Yan H, Wang H, Han Z, Hallahan D (2010) Radiation-guided drug delivery to mouse models of lung cancer. Clin Cancer Res 16 (20):4968–4977

Hariri G, Wellons M, Morris W, Lukehart C, Hallahan D (2011) Multifunctional FePt nanoparticles for radiation-guided targeting and imaging of cancer. Ann Biomed Eng 39(3):946–952

Harris E, Christensen V, Hwang W, Fox K, Solin L (2005) Impact of concurrent versus sequential tamoxifen with radiation therapy in early-stage breast cancer patients undergoing breast conservation treatment. J Clin Oncol 23(1):11–16

Herold D, Das I, Stobbe C, Iyer R, Chapman J (2000) Gold microspheres: a selective technique for producing biologically effective dose enhancement. Int J Radiat Biol 76:1357–1364

Hoffman A (2008) The origins and evolution of "controlled" drug delivery systems. J Controlled Release 132:153–163

Hofheinz R, Gnad-Vogt S, Beyer U, Hochhaus A (2005) Liposomal encapsulated anti-cancer drugs. Anticancer Drugs 16:691–707

Holli K, Hietanen P, Saaristo R, Huhtala H (2009) Radiotherapy after segmental resection of breast cancer with favorable prognostic features: 12-year follow-up results of a randomized trial. J Clin Oncol 27(6):927–932

Horcajada P, Chalati T, Serre C, Gillet B, Sebrie C, Batti T et al (2010) Porous metal-organic-framework nanoscale carries as a potential platform for drug delivery and imaging. Nat Mater 9:172–178

Hughes K, Schnaper L, Berry D (2004) Lumpectomy plus tamoxifen with or without irradiation in women 70 years of age or older with early breast cancer. NEJM 351:971–977

Jamison T, Bakhshi R, Petrova D, Pocock R, Imani M, Seifalian A (2007) Biological applications of quantum dots. Biomaterials 28:4717–4732

Janes K, Fresneau M, Marazuela A, Fabra A, Alonso M (2001) Chitosan nanoparticles as delivery systems for doxorubicin. J Controlled Release 73:255–267

Johannes L, Lamaze C (2002) Clathrin-dependent or not: is it still the question? Traffic 3(7):443–451

Keall P, Arnfield M, Arhtur D (2001) An IMRT technique to reduce the heart and lung dose for early stage breast cancer. Int J Radiat Oncol Biol Phys 51(Suppl 1):247

Keynes G (1937) Conservative treatment of cancer of the breast. Br Med J 2:643–649

Khan F (2003) The physics of radiation therapy, 3rd edn. Lippincott Williams and Wilkins, Philadelphia

Khan M, Minc L, Nigavekar S, Kariapper M, Nair B (2008) Fabrication of 198Au0 radioactive composite nanodevices and their use for nanobrachytherapy. Nanomed Nanotechnol Biol Med 4:57–69

Kievit F, Wang F, Fang C, Mok H, Wang K (2011) Doxorubicin loaded iron oxide overcome multidrug resistence in cancer in vitro. J Controlled Release 152(1):76–83

Kim T, Kim D, Chung J (2004) Phase I and pharmacokinetic study of genexol-PM, a cremophor-free, polymeric micelle-formulated paclitaxel, in patients with advanced malignancies. Clin Cancer Res 10:3708–3716

Kim D, Rozhkova E, Ulasov I, Bader S, Rajh T, Lesniak W et al (2010) Biofunctioalized magnetic-vortex microdiscs for targeted cancer-cell destruction. Nat Mater 9(2):165–171

King T, Bolton J, Kuske R, Fuhrman G, Scroggin T, Jiang X (2000) Long term results of wide-field brachytherapy as the sole method of radiation therapy after segmental mastectomy for T(is, 1, 2) breast cancer. Am J Surg 180:299–304

Kirkham M, Parton R (2005) Clathrin-independent endocytosis: new insights into caveloae and non-caveolar lipid raft carriers. Biochimica et Biophysica Acta 1746(3):349–363

Kong T, Zheng J, Wang X, Yang J, McQuarrie S (2008) Enhancement of radiation cytotoxicity in breast cancer cells by localized attachment of gold nanoparticles. Small 4(9):1537–1543

Koukourakis M, Giatromanolaki A, Pitiakoudis M, Kouklakis G, Tsoutsou P (2010) Concurrent liposomal cisplatin (lipoplatin), 5-fluorouracil and radiotherapy for the treatment of locally advanced gastric cancer: a phase I/II study. Int J Radiat Oncol Biol Phys 78(1):150–155

Kratz F, Drevs J, Bing G, Stockmar C, Scheuermann K (2001) Development and in vitro efficacy of novel MMP2 and MMP9 specific doxorubicin albumin conjugates. Bioorg Med Chem Lett 11:2001–2006

Kukowska-Latallo J, Candido K, Cao Z, Nigavekar S, Majoros I, Thomas T (2005) Nanoparticle targeting of anticancer drug improves therapeutic response in animal model of human epithelial cancer. Cancer Res 65(12):5317–5324

Larrick J, Wright S (1990) Cytotoxic mechanism of tumour necrosis factor-α. FASEB J. 4:3215–3223

Lesniak W, Kariapper M, Nair B, Tan W, Hutson A, Balogh L et al (2007) Synthesis and characterization of PAMAM dendrimer-based multifunctional nanodevices for targeting αvβ3 integrins. Bioconjug Chem 18:1148–1154

Leuschner C, Kumar C, Hansel W, Soboyejo W, Zhou J, Hormes J (2006) LHRH-conjugated magnetic iron oxide nanoparticles for detection of breast cancer metastases. Breast Cancer Res Treat 99:163–176

Li C (2002) Poly(L-glutamic acid)-anticancer drug conjugates. Adv Drug Deliv Rev 54:695–713

Liu C, Wang C, Chien C, Yang T, Chen S, Leng W (2008) Enhanced X-ray irradiation-induced cancer cell damage by gold nanoparticles treated by a new synthesis method of polyethylene glycol modification. Nanotechnology 19:295104

Liu Z, Ran A, Rakhra K, Sherlock S, Goodwin A, Chen X (2009) Supramolecular stacking of doxorubicin on carbon nanotubes for in vivo cancer therapy. Angew Chem Int Ed 48:7668–7672

Loo C, Lowery A, Halas N, West J, Drezek R (2005) Immunotargeted nanoshells or integrated cancer imaging and therapy. Nano Lett 5:709–711

Lowery A, Onishko H, Hallahan D, Han Z (2011) Tumor-targeted delivery of liposome-encapsulated doxorubicin by use of a peptide that selectively binds to irradiated tumors. J Controlled Release 150:117–124

Malam Y, Loizidou M, Seifalian A (2009) Liposomes and nanoparticles: nanosized vehicles for drug delivery in cancer. Trends Pharmacol Sci 30(11):592–599

Malik N, Evagorou E, Duncan R (1999) Dendrimer-platinate: a novel approach to cancer chemotherapy. Anticancer Drugs 10:767–776

Malik N, Wiwattanapatapee R, Klopsch R, Lorenz K, Frey H, Weener J et al (2000) Dendrimers: relationship between structure and biocompatibility in vitro and preliminary studies on the biodistribution of 125-I labelled PAMAM dendrimers in vivo. J Controlled Release 65:133–148

Markman M (2006) Pegylated liposomal doxorubicin in the treatment of cancers of the breast and ovary. Expert Opin Pharmacother 7:1469–1474

Mehta V, Algan O, Grien K (2010) Experience with an electronic brachytherapy technique for intracavitary accelerated partial breast irradiation. Am J Clin Oncol 33(4):327–335

Mello R, Callisen H, Winter J, Kagan A, Norman A (1983) Radiation dose enhancement in tumors with iodine. Med Phys 10:75–78

Menard C, Camphausen K, Muanza T (2003) Clinical trial of endorectal amifostine for radioprotection in patients with prostate cancer: rational and early results. Semin Oncol 30(Suppl. 18):63–67

Mesa A, Norman A, Solberg T, Demarco J, Smathers J (1999) Dose distribution using kilovoltage X-rays and dose enhancement from iodine contrast agents. Phys Med Biol 44:1955–1968

Milele E, Spinelli G, Miele E, Tomao F, Tomao S (2009) Albumin-bound formulation of Paclitaxel (Avraxane® ABI-007) in the treatment of breast cancer. Int J Nanomed 4:99–105

Mille M, Xu G, Rivard M (2010) Comparison of organ doses for patients undergoing balloon brachytherapy of the breast with hdr 192-Ir or electronic sources using monte carlo simulation in a heterogeneous human platform. Med Phys 37(2):662–671

Misawa M, Takahashi J (2011) Generation of reactive oxygen species induced by gold nanoparticles under X-ray and UV irradiations. Nanomed Nanotechnol Biol Med 7:604–614

Moghimi S, Szebeni J (2003) Stealth liposomes and long circulating nanoparticles: critical issues in pharmacokinetics, opsonization and protein binding properties. Prog Lipid Res 42:463–478

Mosesson Y, Mills G, Yarden Y (2008) Derailed endocytosis: an emerging feature of cancer. Nat Rev Cancer 8(11):835–850

Mukerjee P, Bharracharya R, Wang P, Wang L, Basu S (2005) Antiangiogenic properties of gold nanoparticles. Clin Cancer Res 11(9):3530–3534

Murray CB, Kagan CR, Bawendi MG (1995) Self-organization of CdSe nanocrystallites into three-dimensional quantum dot superlattices. Science 270(1335):1338

Neal A, Torr M, Helyer S (1995) Correlation of breast dose heterogeneity with breast size using 3D CT planning and dose-volume histograms. Radiother Oncol 34:210–218

Nel A, Madler L, Velegol D, Xia T, Hoek E, Somasundaran P et al (2009) Understanding biophysicochemical interactions at the nano-bio interface. Nat Mater 8:543–557

Nigavekar S, Sung L, Llanes M, El-Jawahri A, Lawrence T, Becker C (2004) 3H dendrimer nanoparticle organ/tumor distribution. Pharm Res 21(3):476–483

Oliver M, Chen J, Wong E, Van Dyk J, Perera F (2007) A treatment planning study comparing whole breast radiation therapy against conformal, IMRT and tomotherapy for accelerated partial breast irradiation. Radiother Oncol 82(3):317–323

Pamugula S, Kishore S, Rider B (2005) Radioprotection in mice following oral delivery of amifostine nanoparticles. Int J Radiat Biol 81:251–257

Pan B, Cui D, Sheng Y, Ozkan C, Gao F, He R (2007) Dendrimer-modified magnetic nanoparticles enhance efficacy of gene delivery system. Cancer Res 67:8156–8163

Patel K, Li M, Schuh J, Baldeschwieler J (1984) The pharmacological efficacy of a rigid non-phospholipid liposome drug delivery system. Biochim Biophys Acta 797:20–26

Paunesku T, Rajh T, Wiederrecht G, Maser J, Vogt S, Stojicevic N (2003) Biology of TiO$_2$-oligonucleotide nanocomposites. Nat Mater 2:343–346

Perez C, Brady L, Halperin E, Schmidt-Ullrich R (2004) Principles and practice of radiation oncology, 4th edn. Lippincott Williams & Wilkins, Philadelphia

Pierce L, Hutchins L, Green S, Lew D, Gralow J, Livingston R et al (2005) Sequencing of tamoxifen and radiotherapy after breast-conserving surgery in early-stage breast cancer. J Clin Oncol 23(1):24–29

Rabatic B, Dimitrijevic N, Cook R, Saponjic Z, Rajh T (2006) Spatially confined corner defects induce chemical functionality of TiO$_2$ nanorods. Adv Mater 18(8):1033–1037

Rahman W, Bishara N, Ackerly T, He C, Jackson P, Wong C et al (2009) Enhancement of radiation effects by gold nanoparticles for superficial radiation therapy. Nanomed Nanotechnol Biol Med 5:136–142

Recht A (2003) Integration of systemic therapy and radiation therapy for patients with early-stage breast cancer treated with conservative surgery. Clin Breast Cancer 4:104–113

Reed J, Miyashita T, Takayama S, Wang H, Sato T, Krajewski S et al (1996) Bcl-2 family proteins: regulators of cell death in the pathogenesis of cancer and resistance to therapy. J Cell Biochem 60:23–32

Rivera E (2003a) Liposmal anthracyclines in metatstaic breast cancer: clinical update. Oncologist 8(Suppl 2):3–9

Rivera E (2003b) Current status of liposomal antracycline therapy in metastatic breast cancer. Clin Breast Cancer 4:S76–S83

Robar J, Ribbio S, Martin M (2002) Tumour dose enhancement using modified megavoltage photon beams and contrast media. Phys Med Biol 47:2433–2449

Sabbatini P, Aghajanian C, Dizon D (2004) Phase II study of CT-2103 in patients with recurrent epithelial ovarian, fallopian tube, or primary peritoneal carcinoma. J Clin Oncol 22:4523–4531

Schweitzer A, Howell C, Jiang Z (2009) Physico-chemical evaluation of rationally designed melanins as novel nature-inspired radioprotectors. PLoS ONE 4:e7229

Schweitzer A, Revskaya E, Chu P, Pazo V, Friedman M, Nosanchuk J et al (2010) Melanin-covered nanoparticles for protection of bone marrow during radiation therapy of cancer. Int J Radiat Oncol Biol Phys 78(5):1494–1502

Sekhon B, Kamboj S (2010a) Inorganic nanomedicine—part 2. Nanomed Nanotechnol Biol Med 6:612–618

Sekhon B, Kamboj S (2010b) Inorganic nanomedicine—part 1. Nanomed Nanotechnol Biol Med 6:516–522

Sini P, Wyder L, Schnell C, O'Reilly T (2005) The antitumor and antiangiogenic activity of vascular endothelial growth factor receptor inhibition is potentiated by ErbB1 blockade. Clin Cancer Res 11:4521–4532

Small W (2003) Radiation therapy oncology group C-0116 trial. Cytoprotection/radioprotection with amifostine: potential role in cervical cancer and early findings in the radiation therapy oncology group C-0116 trial. Semin Oncol 30(Suppl. 18):68–71

Steinhauser I, Spankuch B, Strebhardt K, Langer K (2006) Trastuzumab-modified nanoparticles: optimisation of preparation and uptake in cancer cells. Biomaterials 27:4975–4983

Tanaka T, Decuzzi P, Cristofanilli M, Sakamoto J, Tasciotti E, Robertson F et al (2009) Nanotechnology for breast cancer therapy. Biomed Microdevices 11:49–63

Taylor-Pashow K, Rocca J, Huxford R, Lin W (2010) Hybrid nanomaterials for biomedical applications. Chem Commun 46: 5832–5849

Tomalia D, Baker J, Dewald M, Hall G, Kallos S, Martin J et al (1985) A new class of polymers: starburst-dendritic macromolecules. Polym J 17:117–132

Tsujimoto Y (1998) Role of Bcl-2 family proteins in apoptosis: apoptosome or mitochondria. Genes Cells 3(11):687–707

Vasey P, Kaye S, Morrison T, Twelves C, Wilson P, Duncan P, Phase I (1999) Clinical and pharmacokinetic study of PK1 [N-(2-hydroxy-propyl)-methacrylaminde copolymer doxorubicin]: first member of a new class of chemotherapeutic agents–drug-polymer conjugates. Clin Cancer Res 5:83–94

Veronesi U, Marubini E, Marian L (2001a) Radiotherapy after breast-preserving surgery in small breast carcinoma: long-term results of a randomized trial. Ann Oncol 12:997–1003

Veronesi U, Oreechia R, Luini A (2001b) A preliminary report of intraoperative radiotherapy (IORT) in limited-stage breast cancers that are conservatively treated. Eur J Cancer 37:2178–2183

Vinci F, Baglan K, Kestin L (2001) Accelerated treatment of breast cancer. J Clin Oncol 19(7):1993–2001

Vivero-Escoto J, Slowing I, Trewyn B, Lin V (2010) Mesoporous silica nanoparticles for intracellular controlled drug delivery. Small 6 (18):1952–1967

Wang A, Yuet K, Zhang L, Gu F, Huynh-Le M (2010) ChemoRad nanoparticles: a novel multifunctional nanoparticle platform for targeted delivery of concurrent chemoradiation. Nanomed 5 (3):361–368 London

Wazer D, Berle L, Graham R (2002) Preliminary results of a phase I/II study of HDR brachytherapy alone for T1/T2 breast cancer. Int J Radiat Oncol Biol Phys 53(4):889–897

Werner M, Copp J, Karve S, Cummings N, Sukumar R, Li C (2011) Folate-targeted polymeric nanoparticle formulation of docetaxel is an effective molecularly targeted radiosensitizer with efficacy dependant on the timing of radiotherapy. ACS Nano 5(11):8990–8998

Wisse E, Braet F, Luo D (1996) Structure and function of sinusoidal lining cells in the liver. Toxicol Pathol 24:100–111

Wu A, Paunesku T, Zhang Z, Vogt S, Lai B, Maser J (2011) A multimodal nanocomposite for biomedical imaging. AIP Conf Proc 1365:379–383

Xie J, Chen K, Huang J, Lee S, Wang J (2010) PET/NIRF/MRI triple functional iron oxide nanoparticles. Biomaterials 31:3016–3022

Yoo H, Oh J, Lee K, Park T (1999) Biodegradable nanoparticles containing doxorubicin-PLGA conjugate for sustained release. Pharm Res 16:1114–1118

Yoo H, Lee K, Oh J, Park T (2000) In vitro and in vivo anti-tumor activities of nanoparticles based on doxorubicin-PLGA conjugates. J Controlled Release 68(3):419–431

Yuan F, Dellian M, Fukumua D (1995) Vascular permeability in the human tumor xenograft: molecular size dependence and cutoff size. Cancer Res 55:3752–3756